A TO Z GUIDE TO PREGNANCY

A HOLISTIC GUIDE FOR YOUR BEAUTIFUL JOURNEY – PREGNANCY

SRUTHY M R

Thank You!

"To my parents Jaya and Rajan who taught me to do good to others. To my soul sister Keerthy who always stood by me. To my husband, Vishnu who constantly motivates me with his love and encouragement to achieve the best with my capability. Above all, my heart goes to the beloved mothers who crossed their journey of motherhood with me on the path called 'Life'! "

Contents

Preface

About the Author

Sruthy Manuvelil Rajan comes with a holistic experience of Clinical, Psychological, and NLP Practices of over twelve years. As a counselor and a writer, she has so far served thousands of adults in the area of health and psyche through her counseling, health coaching and blogging.

During her consultations, Sruthy came across many cases of emotional and health issues arising from pre-birth traumas. She staunchly believes such issues could be averted if people receive ideal education regarding pregnancy and childbirth. 'A to Z guide to Pregnancy' is created with an intention of educating the couples regarding proper care to enhance the birth of a healthy baby.

Disclaimer: *This book is not a substitute for medical consultation, instead, it is a collection of facts and health practices you can adopt during your pregnancy.*

Acknowledgements

I would like to thank:

Keerthy Rajan & Vishnu Raveendran: For designing, editing, and providing critical reviews of this book.

The mothers who cooperated with me during my undergraduate studies for the case studies on normal and abnormal pregnancies, abdominal examinations, and health assessment and monitoring. They are in fact the solid foundation of this book.

Above all, my head bows to my high school teachers; Alex Sir, Jency Sir, my college Principal Sr. Elsy, Vice Principal Mrs. Ammini Poulose, and the Obstetric and Gynaecology teachers, Jayashree, Indu, and Amruta. My NLP Guru, Vikram Dhar, and my personal coach Manu. Thank you for molding me into who I am today.

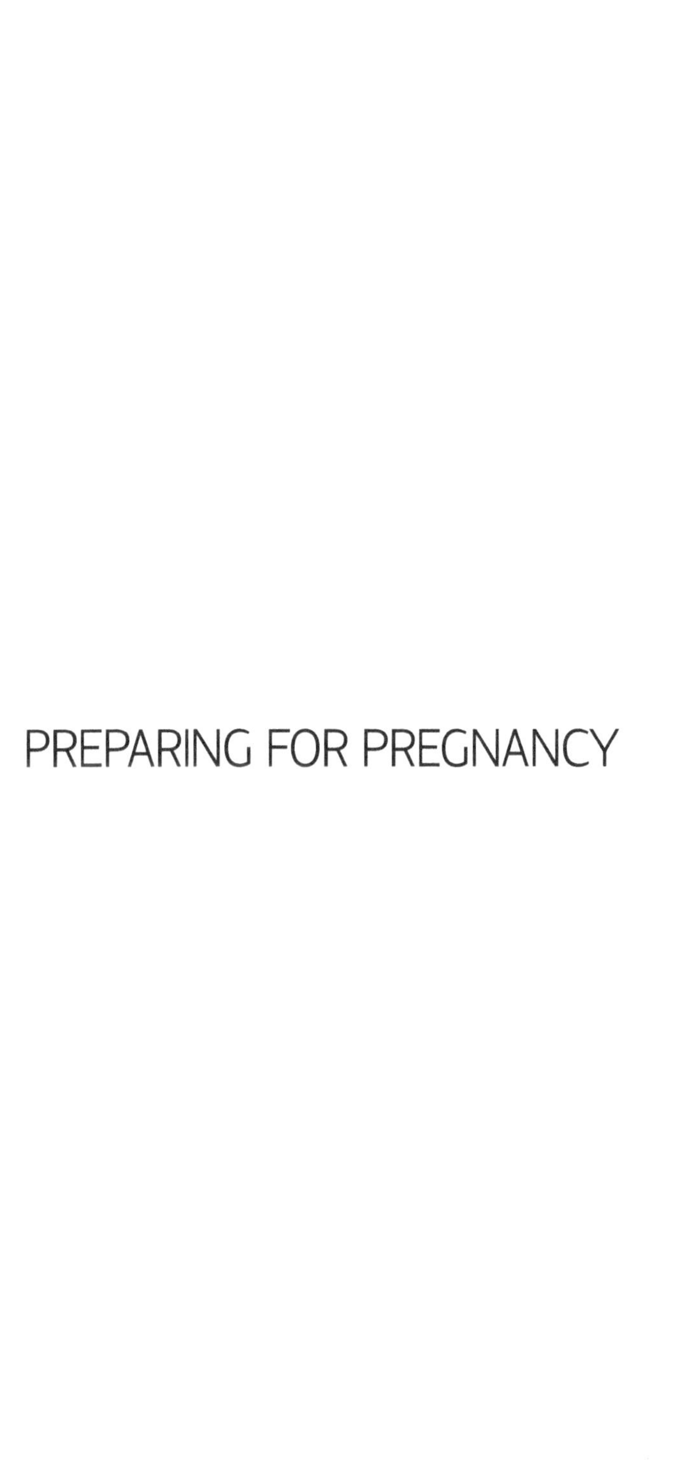

PREPARING FOR PREGNANCY

CHAPTER ONE

Taking Care of your Mind

Thinking of having a new member in your life? Well, your mind can go through a lot of places when you imagine pregnancy! From those morning sicknesses to the routine medical checkups and aching legs, both of you couples might probably get exhausted and thus have already created a negative picture about pregnancy when in reality, it's not!

Preparing your mind for the possible adaptations for the pregnancy can have amazing results in your journey all through the 9 months! You might probably consider talking to your mother, family members, or even friends who have already gone through childbearing and obviously childbirth!

Another way of familiarising pregnancy is to attend antenatal classes or simply subscribe to free online classes for expectant mothers and of course, read this book! Each time your mind acquaintances with the concept of conception, it gives out a sigh in big relief because at last, you are befriending the so-called negative or fearful thought of 'pregnancy'.

Once you are mentally accommodating 'pregnancy', your body will automatically long for the basic instinct of motherhood.

You will subconsciously lookout for circumstances to get pregnant such as having intercourse on one of your most fertile days (See the FAQ for the Fertility Cycle), developing a special like for the food that enhances your sexual urge. This will ultimately result in enhancing your fertility and you will adapt to whatever state possible to grow a young one inside you!

Now, how can you take proper care of your mind in such a way that you stay completely optimistic about pregnancy? There are ways for this too! Think about your favorite hobby and start with it! Considering going for a 15 minutes walk or spending your free time in the greens. All these positive activities can help you cleanse your mind. An additional recommendation is to join a Yoga class and practice it in the morning. Giving thought to traveling can be an excellent idea too! Some people stay positive by joining laughing clubs or simply watching funny videos as well!

And finally, meditation is also another magnificent method to sanitize your mind! Throughout this book, you can find several mentions and meditation techniques described for the same reason. However, you can choose your favorite method of meditation. This can vary from a silent one to fishing and even a bathing meditation. The point is to feel calm and to be aware of the present.

Having explained about the nutrients for your mind, I would like to add up the 'no - no's for your brain too! They are: Stay away from toxic people in your life Stop engaging in gossip and bad talk about people Rather than thinking of not wanting anything, think of what you want Forget the word 'complaining' and start the habit of gratitude Once your mind brims with positivism, it starts reflecting on your body too. Being positive, you can find the breaths you take to be fresher and life itself starts to take a beautiful turn all for you! What an amazing start it would be for your pregnancy! To give birth to a baby from a body with alluring enthusiasm!

CHAPTER TWO

Your Mind Matters!

In the previous chapter, we equipped our bodies to prepare for the pregnancy. As goes the famous adage, half begun is well done, your body will automatically shift its gear towards your becoming pregnant if you feel ready for it with all senses. But how about a few tips that can help you to find perfection in the health statement?

Several factors aid in enhancing your fertility and in turn childbirth. Hence it's crucial to scrutinize each one.

1. Body Mass Index (BMI) and Fertility

An ideal *BMI for childbearing is found to be around 23. Overweight or Underweight are found to be riskier for pregnancy as there are more chances of fetal damage and stunted growth in babies. However, your genetic body type can be an exception. For instance, if you are slim from the beginning (like your mother's or father's body type) and did not lose weight due to your lifestyle or any disease you may safely undergo childbearing and childbirth. The same goes when you are a little over the desired body weight as well.

***BMI CALCULATION**

There are many online BMI Calculators available online on Google.

2. Body Fat

Several pieces of research reveal that increased fat distribution around the abdomen, as opposed to the hips and thighs, is associated with reduced chances of conception. You might also note that the body fat increases if you do not exercise, experience stress, or suffer from any metabolic disorders such as Hypothyroidism* or any emotional or psychological issues such as Depression, Stress, or Anxiety.

***Hypothyroidism:** The condition in which your thyroid gland doesn't produce enough of certain crucial hormones. *Gestational Diabetes & Hypertension: A type of diabetes & Hypertension that can develop during pregnancy in women who don't already have diabetes and/or high blood pressure. *Fetal Macrosomia: A newborn baby who is much larger than the average.

3. Nutritional Status

A well-nourished diet is crucial for both partners once the plan of conception pops up in your mind. Because most of the organogenesis (formation of organs) of the embryo* takes place in the initial stage, even before the couple finds out they are expecting a baby, it is always safer to be prepared and provide a congenial environment for the baby to grow.

While the underweight or malnourished mothers are likely to give birth to babies with low birth weight and growth retardation, overweight or obese mothers are more prone to develop gestational diabetes* and hypertension*. Pregnant women with obesity have higher chances of Cesarean delivery and *fetal macrosomia

4. Exercises and Optimization of Body Weight

It is an indisputable fact that you can very well have spontaneous ovulation and conception when a program of regular exercises and weight loss are adhered to. Similarly, improving your health by resorting to physical exercises of at least 30 minutes a day (this does not include your household chores, yes, what I mean here is a dedicated half an hour workout) will make you fit for conception.

5. Eating a Balanced Diet

It is desirable to eat more starchy foods such as cereals and bread, at least five portions of fruit and vegetables daily, and less fatty foods. Healthy eating is not always easy on a limited budget. Foods such as baked beans, jacket potatoes, sardines, and tuna are relatively cheap but nutritious. It is also important to carefully watch out if you have any allergies to any food items or if you newly develop one during pregnancy. For the latter, I suggest you refrain from eating a new item; but if you cannot resist the temptation, go for a smaller quantity first and proceed if no adverse reaction occurs. Maintaining an ideal BMI, eating the right foods, and performing regular exercises are applicable to both partners to make sure they have a healthy conception. This helps minimize the number of risks during your labor as well. The more you are good at these, the more beneficial it is for your baby.

CHAPTER THREE

The Four Pillars of Fertility

Forming a definite platform for conception is crucial as this helps to ensure the organogenesis of your baby is governed in the right way. There are 4 essential components that determine your fertility and fetal well-being.

1. Vitamin E

While the exact role of this fat-soluble vitamin is still unknown, this plays a significant role in enhancing your fertility. This vitamin is seen in abundance in foods such as nuts, seeds, and vegetable oils. Ensure you include almonds, spinach, avocado, and squashes in your daily diet.

2. Omega 3 Fatty Acids

These are the good fats that help in the development of your baby's nervous system. As mentioned earlier, the primitive form of the nervous system develops as early as 3 weeks. It is crucial to stock in some of these nutrients well before in advance. The deficiency of this component is found to be the cause of *birth defects or *neural tube defects (NTDs) in children.

***Birth Defects:** Birth defects are structural changes present at birth that can affect almost any part or parts of the body.

***Neural Tube Defect:** Neural tube defects are severe birth defects of the brain and spine.

If you consume non-vegetarian food, dietary sources like fish (especially seawater fishes like Sardine and Tuna), prawns, mussels, and crabs would supplement you with the required Omega 3 Fatty Acids. It is wise to rule out mercury poisoning when you consume fish such as tuna and salmon. However, if you are a vegan or you are expecting at an elderly age (that is, both or any of you are over 30 years of age), I advocate a Gynaecologist's advice for taking supplementary capsules that usually comes as over the counter ones like 'Seacod' fish oil. You may find the medicine your doctor prescribed bears 'DHA' in it. Docosahexaenoic Acid (DHA)is a type of Omega 3 fat.

3. Folic Acid

Folic acid or Vitamin B9 is an essential component when you plan to conceive. It catalyzes the production of new cells, especially the red blood cells* (RBCs) in our body. While Folic acid is essential for our day-to-day life, it is important to ensure your adequate intake before conception. Seek advice from your family doctor or a Gynaecologist on taking Folic Acid. Although in India Folic Acid tablets are available without a prescription, I have seen almost 100% of the doctors prescribing them to pregnant women during their initial visit to the clinic.

The medicine is available free of cost in the Indian Primary Health Care Centres as well. Lack of this vitamin is associated with birth defects.

4. Vitamin A

A group of compounds such as retinal, retinol, and carotenoids constitutes this Vitamin. The main functions of this Vitamin include growth and development, enhancing the immune system, and helping in vision. The right amount of Vitamin A during pregnancy is associated with birth defects and/ or death rates and vision defects such as night blindness in children. It is equally important to notice that an excess of this component proves to be malignant to the baby as it can cause vision loss. While food such as fish oils, milk, eggs, oranges, and green leafy vegetables can yield retinol, it is judicious to avoid liver and liver products before 3 months of your pregnancy. Many incidences are also reported in developed countries where enormous consumption of foods rich in Vitamin A caused permanent vision disorders in babies.

Modifying your Lifestyle

Apart from the mind and body, lifestyle modification is also needed to make your preparation for pregnancy complete! Here are the simple ways you can adopt to ensure you stay healthy inside out while you get ready to invite that new partner into your life!

Start and End your Day with Meditation

Meditating is an excellent idea for keeping yourself on track for the rest of the day! You just have to spend 5 minutes at the very start and end of the day. This gives you a sense of awareness which enables you to understand your likes and dislikes as well. For example, you might be drinking all day just to escape from the work pressure without giving it much thought that it could be harmful to your conception. With meditation, you become increasingly aware of your addictive habits and thus pose a greater chance to find out healthy alternatives for drinking!

Meditating is an excellent idea for keeping yourself on track for the rest of the day! You just have to spend 5 minutes at the very start and end of the day. You just have to spend 5 minutes at the very start and end of the day. This gives you a sense of awareness which enables you to understand your likes and dislikes as well.

For example, you might be drinking all day just to escape from the work pressure without giving it much thought that it could be harmful to your conception. With meditation, you become increasingly aware of your addictive habits and thus pose a greater chance to find out healthy alternatives for drinking! I wish to guide you to a simple meditation that you can perform sitting anywhere, even in your bed. For best results, include your partner as well! You can include soothing music as the background if you wish to.

Meditation Steps

"Meditation means dissolving the invisible walls that unawareness has built ." - **Sadhguru**

- Find a place where you are unlikely to be disturbed Sit with your legs folded (Sukhasana) and eyes closed Start taking small breaths and eventually make them deeper and slower
- Let your thoughts soar at first.
- Do not stop them Now imagine a small baby.
- And you are holding it, enjoying its plays, the giggles.
- Visualize it is holding your fingers with its tiny grasp.
- You are still keeping eye contact with it.
- Feel the feeling of pure joy and happiness.
- You know nothing on earth is worrying you now as you're immersed in the pure joy
- Be in the moment for as long as you wish
- Now slowly concentrate on your breaths. Notice the air going in and out Open your eyes and smile (at your partner if present)

See your baby wherever you want to see it!

Decorate your bedroom with those cute hangings just like you want it to be if you had a baby! Paste in some cute pictures of a baby in your room or laptop or wherever you feel like seeing it. Watch baby movies and see some of the funny videos of kids!

If you love cooking, make some funny dishes with popping eyes and colorful dishes just like you would do if you had a kid. If you are a private person, do it when you're alone!

For the daddies to be, find some time for playing games with kids who stays around you! Imbibe their young spirit and think of nothing but pure pleasure when you are with them. Imagine you are playing this game with your own kid (even if you are not seeing it physically!)

Indulge yourself in them by all means and you will see your body getting ready by all means to receive the young one in no time!

However, it is important not to focus on your thoughts on any negative feelings associated with pregnancy whenever you see those images. You might be going through tough times already, like your family members forcing you to have a kid soon.

You may also have experienced an unfortunate incident like losing someone special recently. History of abortions or miscarriages may also shake your confidence to conceive with happiness. All of these might bring both partners' energy down.

Practicing daily mindfulness would increase your awareness whereby you can readily identify that your 'inability' or 'delay' in conception is not your fault, instead all you can do is to accept, acknowledge and be optimistic despite the history.

Having said that, you may now close this book for a while to find some cute images of babies to put on your Mobile, Laptop, or anywhere in your room or house!

Eat better!

Eating healthier food is essential to make sure you are fit. Unfortunately, we are left with fewer choices to eat good foods. Where organic foods are found to be expensive anywhere in the world, finding the right food within your budget can be challenging

You still have hope though! Resorting to eat local fruits and vegetables can be a good option. They are less likely to be unhealthy compared to the instant foods or processed foods that you get from the supermarkets.

You can consider creating tiny gardens in your kitchen or backyard or even in your apartment! Thanks to the internet you can find infinite ways just by browsing in your free time.

Avoiding junk foods can be another challenge to overcome. But here's the catch! There is a principle that applies to every human being. The principle of 'pain and pleasure.' We associate pain with some activity and hence try to avert that. And cling on to the activity which pleases our mind.

Similarly, imagine the healthy food you eat is going to benefit your child be born and that you are in an active role to make your child a healthy one in the future. I bet, all of us want to be responsible parents, wouldn't we? Think of all the metabolic disorders we suffer now as the result of man's greed to gulp in those artificial foods! Now link the pleasure of creating your healthy kid to the 'good foods' and pain with the picture of a kid who falls sick occasionally because of its low immunity! There you are, the challenge is solved!

Work Hard to Work Out

This is my favorite suggestion for your couples! Our cells rejuvenate and repair all by themselves. Components such as good thoughts (gives positivity), good foods (gives nutrients for the building process), and physical activity (accelerates the process of becoming 'new') is needed to make sure the process of rejuvenation is at optimum.

This suggestion becomes prominent when your age is over 30. For various reasons, cell division and cell growth stunt (unless you're a person who has a very good lifestyle). Hence it is advisable to include an exercise routine in your life.

There are numerous ways to burn calories with fun. It is best if you include a set of 12 Sun Salutations in the morning. But for beginners, it is all right to start with 2 to 4 sets of the same. In addition to this, perform 10 minutes of moderate to heavy workouts depending on your physical health. Those who are adrenaline junkies can go out and seek nature's adventure through trekking or kayaking instead of indoor workouts!

The dancers can dance to the beat of reggae or hip hop, the tennis lovers can enjoy their time with the sport or the swimmers can find a great time swimming in the water! You just have to choose the type of workout close to your heart!

Adopting a healthy lifestyle creates a sense of happiness and responsibility for one's own life. The happier you are, the more it reflects on each of your life's arenas! What else would be the best preparation for pregnancy than you both becoming the perfect daddy and mommy for your kid!

From Month 1 to 9 and Some More or Less!

CHAPTER FIVE

Pregnancy Simplified

The pregnancy journey begins when one of those 300 million sperm meets the ovum in the uterine tube. The membrane of the ovum is sealed soon after the penetration and now we have 2 nuclei in a single cell (one from the sperm and another from the ovum). The fertilized ovum is thus called a Zygote.

The life span of both the sperm and ovum is not more than 2 or 3 days and hence fertilization (union of sperm and ovum) is likely to occur when intercourse takes place about 14 days before the next period is due.

The 'Living Ball' turned into a baby

When the little ball aka the ovum is fertilized, it rolls down to the uterus and starts further cell division. First, it divides into 2 cells, then into 4, then 8,16, and so on until a mulberry-shaped 'morula' is formed.

Next, a fluid-filled cavity called 'blastocele' appears in the morula, together the fluid and mass are called 'blastocyst'. Around this 'fluid and mass' ball, another layer called 'trophoblast' forms. Later the trophoblast becomes the placenta and the cell mass and fluid become the baby and the amniotic fluid respectively.

Before you name your baby, it gets a couple of names (Viz blastocele, trophoblast, etc) right from the moment life begins to emerge in it!

Zygote - The fertilized ovum formed by the fusion of sperm and ovum. The name remains until it completes 3 weeks.

Embryo - Starting from 3 weeks until 8, the cell mass is called an embryo.

Foetus - Once the life form grows further (from the 8th week onwards), it is called a 'fetus' or 'baby' until birth.

Both your body and the baby undergo growth, adaptations, and transformations throughout pregnancy. In the following chapters, you will understand how your body equips so wonderfully!

CHAPTER SIX

Growth and Development of the Baby

Your baby gets nourishment through the placenta, the organ that the mother's body develops on its own! The nutrients present in your blood go through this organ. From the placenta, it reaches the fetus through the umbilical cord. This cord is inserted through the umbilicus (or the belly button) and hence the name.

From day one, your baby never rests until the term when most of the organs and their functions are established. A series of development occur in your baby's growth and development.

0 to 4 weeks after conception

- Rapid growth
- Primitive central nervous system forms
- The heart develops and begins to beat
- Limb buds form

Your Food & Nutrition

- Eat nutrient-rich foods
- Ensure adequate hydration
- Ensure your mental well being while you eat - Eat with peace at a peaceful place
- Eat health supplements as directed by your consultant

Foods to Avoid

Pineapple, Papaya, Peach, Litchi, Aloe vera, Drumstick or any products from the Drumstick tree, Coffee (you can use it in moderation if not at all avoidable), Green Tea, Soft Cheese (made from unpasteurized milk), Smoked and Tinned fish and meat, Cold Cuts, Canned fruit juice.

Activities

- Avoid strenuous activities
- No alcohol and smoking
- Take regular walks

Medication

- Regulate your drug dosage
- Do not take Over - The - Counter drugs (OTC Drugs) or any medicines or preparations upon referral of a layperson or your fellow friend or relative or social media ads without the consultation of a specialist

4 to 8 weeks after conception

- Very rapid cell division
- Head and facial features develop
- All major organs are in the primitive form
- Early movements Visible on ultrasound from 6 weeks

Your Food & Nutrition

- Have a basic health check-up and start supplementary medicines as per the prescription
- Ensure Calcium, Mineral, and Vitamin-rich nutrition
- Go rainbow!!! - Consume vegetables and greens with varied colors.
- Try picking those violet and green colored aubergines (eggplant or brinjal), golden yellow squashes, or colored bell peppers (popularly known in India as Capsicum).
- You may have more Fruit Juices of your choice Alternatives for fruit juices are skimmed milk, Coconut water, Rice water, or clarified buttermilk

Special Concern

- Continue Basic Blood tests and /or check-ups
- You may develop an urge to Urinate
- May experience Constipation
- You might feel Tiredness
- You might also be dealing with an emotional dilemma regarding pregnancy and childbirth

8 to 12 weeks after conception

- Your baby's Eyelids fuse
- Kidneys begin to function and the fetus passes urine from 10 weeks
- Fetal circulation functions properly
- Sucking and swallowing begin Sex is apparent

Your Food & Nutrition

- Consume ghee and honey, especially in the early morning
- Oranges are your baby's skin. Provided you are not experiencing acidity, go ahead and consume fresh oranges or Mosambi (sweet lemon) juice
- For those cute hairs on your baby's head, eat potassium-rich foods such as banana and eggplant
- Continue to hydrate your body by drinking plain water

Assuming you do not have any allergy to seafood, I advise taking iodine-rich food during this time. Some of them are:

- Oysters
- Mussels
- Squids
- Shrimps
- And food cooked in iodized salt or fortified

You require a little more focus on the protein part. You may consider eating protein-rich foods such as :

- Protein shakes
- Salads with sprouts
- Meat and/or Meat Products

Caution:

- Wash vegetables thoroughly
- Ensure the food you eat is cooked well No burnt meat
- Avoid the tempting overburnt grills or charcoal smoke from the restaurants serving smoked meat

Special Concern

Fainting

Be Careful while performing daily activities Use anti-skid footwear Perform Activities with mild to moderate speed Repeat the mantra, "No hurry." Caution while getting up from the bed.

Skin Care

Start applying turmeric – coconut oil paste over your tummy! You can substitute with other prescribed ayurvedic oils for coconut oil that might contain therapeutic ingredients for your skin Wash it off with a natural exfoliant such as green gram powder or basin powder or freshly prepared homemade paste of overnight soaked green gram or chana.

Momnesia (Forgetfulness during pregnancy)

Fix permanent positions for your things Seek your partner's help to support and reassure you when you feel overwhelmed Stick to-do lists, mobile alarms, or a small notebook to keep yourself on track

12 to 16 weeks after conception

- Quickening - Mother feels the fetal movements
- A waxy coating (Vernix caseosa*) is present over the baby inside
- Fingernails can be seen
- Skin cells begin to be renewed

Your Food & Nutrition

Consume plenty of foods rich in Iron, Vitamin C, Protein, Calcium and fiber, and fatty acids

Eat more:

- Whole grains

- Beans
- Lentils
- Legumes
- Dairy products
- Fishes
- Lean meats
- Eggs
- Dried fruits

Tip

- Consume milk along with dried fruits to calm the heat generated in the body
- Have at least 12 glasses of water a day

Special Concern

- Practice regular meditation, mindfulness moments, and/ or prayers for a baby with strong
- Emotional Intelligence (EI)
- For leg cramps, perform foot and leg exercises.
- Elevate your foot whenever seated

20 to 24 weeks after conception

- Most organs become capable of functioning
- Periods of sleep and activity
- Respond to sound
- Skin red and wrinkled

Your Food & Nutrition

- Eat iron-rich foods for your baby's proper development

- Ensure adequate calcium and magnesium for the baby's strong bones and muscles
- Consume Vitamin C and folic acid-rich foods for your baby's metabolic processes

Special Concern

Body Changes

You can expect your body to be additionally putting up to 13 Kilograms extra

Breast Changes

Your breasts might develop 'Colustrum' or the first milk Poach this liquid with a clean tissue Wear supportive bra

Frequent Urination

Drink an adequate amount of water to replenish your body Wear cotton panties to avoid irritation on your private parts

Constipation

Ensure proper fiber intake Take a daily ten to fifteen minutes walk

Skin Care

Have an oil bath at least twice a week Apply a mild moisturizer

Managing Heartburn and Regurgitation

Avoid spicy and fatty foods Elevate your head and upper body with cushions or pillows

Activities

- Move more slowly
- Ensure grip while walking
- Avoid heavy workouts

24 to 28 weeks after conception

- The baby's survival may be expected if born
- Eyelids open
- Respiratory movements

Your Food and Nutrition

Continue taking foods rich in calcium, vitamins, and minerals.

Special Concern

Back Pain

Use comfort measures such as cushions on your back, legs, etc. Do not stand for a prolonged period of time

Leg Cramp

Consume warm milk and fluids Perform foot and leg exercises

Faster Heart Beat

Keep calm Practice relaxation techniques such as meditation

Itching

Apply natural emollients or mild creams. A good option is applying coconut oil or taking an oil bath every alternate day and washing it off with natural exfoliants (such as green gram or basin flour)

Tip for a Happy Baby!

- Listen to music especially instrumental one's Mom, choose your thoughts wisely – think good!
- Daddy read a story for your baby! Laugh loud!

28 to 32 weeks after conception

- Begins to store fat and iron
- Testes descend into the scrotum
- Small hair (Lanugo) disappears from the face

- Skin becomes paler and less wrinkled

Your Food and Nutrition
Concentrate on Iron-rich food.
Consume:

- More seeds and vegetables
- Meat and Poultry

Iron and Vitamin C
For better absorption of iron, have:
Vitamin C rich foods:

- Lemon
- Orange
- Melon

For Protein for your baby's cells and hair, include:

- Chicken
- Pulses
- Sprouts salad

Magnesium for your baby's bones and muscles:

- Almonds
- Pumpkin seeds

Activities

- Need a baby with more alertness? Read books!
- Listen to your favorite music (No rap and heavy rock please!)

Special Concern
Seek immediate medical advice if you:

- Find bleeding at any time
- Experience cramps
- Diminished activity of your baby

32 to 36 weeks after conception

- Increased fat makes the body more rounded
- Small hair (Lanugo) disappears from the body
- Head hair lengthens
- Nails reach the tips of fingers

Your Food and Nutrition

- Consume small frequent meals
- Ensure adequate intake of Carbohydrates and Protein

Have a look at the recommendation below:
Healthy Carbs

- Wholegrains
- Legumes
- Sweet potatoes

Super Protein

- Egg
- Fish
- Soy products
- Lean meat

Good Fats

- Dried fruits
- Skimmed milk

Friendly Fibre

- green leafy
- vegetables
- fruits
- diary products

Special Concern
Clothing

- Wear light-colored clothes
- Avoid red and black dresses

Relax more

- Small walks
- Breathing exercises

36 to 40 weeks after conception

- The term is reached and birth is due
- Contours rounded
- Skull firm

Your Food and Nutrition

- Continue taking a nutritious rich diet
- Ensure adequate nutrition

Consume happy foods

- Chocolate
- Banana
- Passion fruit
- Locally available sweets

Special Concern

- Seek medical help to induce labor
- Your baby is still safe during this period, hence maintain your calm and follow Doctor's advice!

Month of relief

Most of your discomfort or issues tend to disappear or reduce

Knowledge of the growth and development of your young one equips you to take in proper food and modulate activities accordingly. This again helps a mother to be to have an extra eye on the essential nutrients that are indispensable for the baby in order to avoid any birth defects or delays in the intrauterine milestone.

CHAPTER SEVEN

Your Body Changes During Pregnancy

Pregnancy brings more miracles to your body by adapting to a lot of changes to support the growth of your baby in addition to preparing you for lactation post-childbirth.

We will see each change in detail and this will help you to understand why things are different with you as you near your labor. Understanding your body will enable you to adapt to the changes in a better way and feel positive throughout the period.

Uterus

Before pregnancy, the uterus is a small organ located in your pelvic cavity weighing not more than 60 g. But as the pregnancy progresses, it gradually enlarges to accommodate the baby and the associated organs supporting its growth (placenta and amniotic fluid) begin to emerge. This means your uterus weighs as much as 1000 g by the end of your term!

Likewise, the size of the uterus also matters. From its original pear shape, it becomes more globular and rounded.

The change is somewhat similar in almost all the pregnant women and they are observed to be the following:

10th week - Uterus is about the size of an orange

12th week - It grows to the size of a grapefruit (in Hindi - Chakotara)

16th week - It reaches the midway between your belly button and pubic bone (the front part of your pelvic joint)

20th week - The uterus reaches the level of your belly button

30th week - The uterus could be located the midway between the belly button (umbilicus*) and breast bone (xiphisternum*)

38th week - It reaches the level of the breast bone - The uterus reaches the level of your belly button

Heart

Naturally, you develop a sense of warmth and love during your pregnancy. I cannot be wrong if I call you a lady with a big heart, can I? I mean it because your heart enlarges by about 12% of its original size during pregnancy! The sole purpose of its enlargement is to cater to the extra demand of meeting your baby's growth! In addition to this, the uterus and breasts also receive a considerable amount of blood supply for their nourishment.

Blood

The blood volume also expands from 30 to 50%. This is to protect the mother and fetus and meet the demand of the uterus to perform its function. The extra volume also helps in meeting the 'growing' demands of the fetus. It also compensates for the blood loss from the mother's body during childbirth. In addition to the volume, several other changes occur in its composition during pregnancy. Changes in your plasma volume, iron, clotting factors, and antibodies strive to get ready to nurture the growing life inside you!

Respiratory System

The respiratory system consists of two lungs, the diaphragm, and the rib cages. As the pregnancy advances, the enlarging uterus elevates the diaphragm further up. The rib cages are also displaced upwards and outwards.

As the diaphragm pushes the lungs upwards, its capacity is reduced by 5%. Several changes in respiration also occur to make sure the growing fetus gets an adequate amount of oxygen. To ensure this, your respiration becomes much deeper and slow during pregnancy.

Urinary System

The urinary bladder and the ureters are located just in front of the uterus. During pregnancy, the growing uterus puts considerable pressure on both. The bladder capacity is reduced and the ureters are compressed further as the pregnancy advances. The kidneys too enlarge due to the effect of hormones in pregnancy. The increased blood volume also increases the kidneys' workload to produce more urine.

Gastrointestinal System

Pregnancy brings dramatic changes to all of the organs associated with digestion. Your gums become more spongy and soft because of the effect of estrogen. You may have excess production of saliva while you conceive.

The development of new likes and dislikes towards food is quite common during pregnancy so are the cravings! Generally, you can eat food from any particular food group unless it is restricted if you suffer from any endocrine or other disorders. Though it is uncommon to eat non-food substances (Pica*), it is advisable to seek necessary steps as this will interfere with digestion. You might experience an increase or decrease in your thirst and appetite as well.

The displacement of the stomach and intestine by the enlarging uterus also worsen the symptom of indigestion and nausea or vomiting during pregnancy.

Dilatation of the gastroesophageal sphincter (more details in the FAQs) adds up to one of the reasons for throwing up during pregnancy. Marked reduction in bowel movement also occurs in pregnancy which causes constipation. Several studies have shown that the liver and gallbladder may increase in their size and hence abnormal levels of liver enzymes are evident during the blood check-up in pregnancy.

A considerable amount of changes take place in the carbohydrate, protein, and fat metabolism during pregnancy. These processes are accelerated to support the growth and development of the fetus. This calls for an extra intake of food all through the months of your conception. An estimate of 200 Kcal per day is required to meet the growing demand for nurturing your baby. However, this can vary on an individual basis.

Metabolism

Endocrine System

Pregnancy introduces you to a heap of hormones that tirelessly work to sustain the pregnancy until your term. They also help in inducing labor by expelling the baby once it hits the maturation phase.

Skin

The profound effect of hormones such as progesterone and estrogen accounts for the skin's darkening during pregnancy. A dark line runs from the umbilicus to the above called 'linea nigra' appears while you conceive. It is obvious for the stretch marks to arrive during this time. Hormones and weight gain cause the marks which can remain permanently as a mark of pregnancy.

Several other changes such as itching, the appearance of rashes, overgrowing hair, mild hirsutism, and visible tiny blood vessels are common during pregnancy.

Breast

As the pregnancy progresses, your breast undergoes a series of changes. You may experience tingling, painful, or numb sensations as they begin to grow in size for the preparation to lactate your baby! When you near your term, your nipples become prominent and the breast milk can be expressed from your breasts.

Maternal weight

The whole preparation of childbearing accounts for the weight gain during your conception. This can be up to 12.5 Kilograms. The majority of the weight gain is due to the growing fetus, placenta, and amniotic fluid while the blood and body fluids, fat tissues, and the weight of breasts and uterus account for the remaining weight.

I believe by this time you will be amazed at what wonders your body can do for your baby right? Now that you are familiar with the body changes we will see the common symptoms associated with the pregnancy and how to tackle them effectively in the next chapter.

CHAPTER EIGHT

Common Ailments and their during Pregnancy

Abdominal pain

Abdominal pain during pregnancy is a common complaint in pregnancy. The major causes are indigestion and muscle stretching. However, if the pain is sharp accompanied by vaginal bleeding, you should immediately refer to a health care practitioner.

The management of abdominal pain depends on the cause of pain. If you experience indigestion pain, managing the same would give you relief while if the pain is caused by muscle stretching, rest and exercises will prove beneficial for you. (Please refer to Chapter 9 for exercises).

Anemia

The increased demand for blood for the nourishment of your baby might land you in iron deficiency or anemia. The medical condition can also be due to the dilution of iron in the blood that increases its volume during pregnancy!

Having anemia may make you feel light-headed, and nauseated in addition to giving you those panting breaths when you use the stairs!

While mild anemia is common in pregnancy, the following foods will put your body at ease:

- Green vegetables, especially fresh salads
- Cereals like ragi, and oats,
- Indian gooseberries in any form, preferably fresh or as freshly prepared chutneys
- Meat and meat products except for liver (and its products)

Practicing yoga and meditation can replenish your lungs with plenty of Oxygen well enough to supply your body. This can also help relieve the symptoms of anemia.

Back Pain

The growing Uterus pushes back all your internal organs and this process is at its peak when you near your term. Also softening of joints and ligaments to enable smooth childbirth will make your body more fragile and painful. It is therefore important to take proper care of yourself during pregnancy.

Managing back pain is best done through adopting correct posture and the following steps:

- Perform pelvic tilt (Explained in Chapter 9 - Exercises)
- Support your back with comfort measures such as a cushion or a pillow Avoid tight-fitting clothes and shoes stop wearing high heels
- Do not lift/ handle heavy objects Seek advice from your healthcare provider/ health coach for the exercise best suited for your body
- Ensure adequate nutrition and make sure your blood results show normal Calcium and Vitamin D levels
- Perform regular exercises/ yoga even from the days of your family planning

Bleeding Gums

I hope you remember in the previous chapter when I mentioned those swollen gums because of the hormone estrogen's effect. So now your guess is precise! Your gums bleed because of the very same reason! For some mothers to be, Diabetes can predispose them to gum bleeding. In some cases, dental caries (damage to the dental cavity) are reported during pregnancy as well.

Now let's see how can tackle gum bleeding and save a smile on your face always!

- Regular flossing
- Use herbal sticks as a toothbrush at night
- Gargling with lukewarm water with salt dissolved in it
- Adequate hydration
- Drinking citrous fruit juice (provided you have no acidity issues)
- Crunching carrot and cucumber as your snacks

Blurred Vision

By this time you might be familiar with the phenomena of the 'blood shift' to your tummy all for your baby, isn't it? You might experience blurred vision accompanied by dizziness as your brain gets less amount of blood during pregnancy.

Unless you suffer from Preeclampsia* or Gestational Diabetes Mellitus, the temporary disturbance in your vision is common and hence nothing special is required to manage this issue. However, having gripped carpets and sandals at home can safeguard you from those accidental slips when you ambulate.

Breast tenderness

You may experience a tingling sensation, pain, or numbness in your breasts as the pregnancy progresses. And by the second trimester, your breasts can gush out some milk with the mere sight of a baby or its cry! These all are your body's preparation to equip you for breastfeeding post-childbirth.

Following the tips can give you relief from the above symptoms:

- Shift to a supportive bra for supporting your enlarged/engorged breasts
- Gently massage your breasts with mildly heated oil (preferably coconut oil) before bath
- Use a sponge bra to absorb your breast milk (but make sure to wipe them clean often)

Breathlessness

You might be familiar with the phenomena of breathlessness during pregnancy from the life of your friends, relatives, and the tell tales of your colleagues I believe! But unlike them, you are much more knowledgeable and have more awareness because you read the changes in your body (and in your respiratory system) in the previous chapter, isn't it?

Tackling dyspnoea or breathlessness is indeed a challenge, but try the tips below to find relief. But I tell you, it will be a whole lot of relief when you approach your labor. You can breathe in more comfortably as the baby moves down as your delivery date nears!

Here are my tips!

- Practice relaxation exercises daily
- Keep to your left when you lie down
- Provide support while you lie down with a pregnancy pillow (as your pregnancy progresses)

- Eat light meals about 5 to 6 times rather than consuming large portions at single times
- Enjoy a morning walk of 15 minutes in the Sun (preferably in the early morning)

Constipation

Constipation is another common symptom in your pregnancy. The relaxation of your gut creates this issue but let's see what all can be done to have a smooth bowel function!

- Have a 15 minutes early morning walk
- Ensure adequate hydration by drinking plenty of water
- The more fiber-rich food you consume, the better your bowel emptying would be
- Consuming natural husk and ghee would act as stool softeners and hence can be of your help

Fainting

Fainting or dizziness or lightheadedness can be due to various reasons as your body is more concentrating on bringing up a healthy baby! The hormonal effect, blood changes, and variation in heart-pumping can whirl your world to fainting!

While dizziness is common and (profound) in most first pregnancies, you can be relieved when it's your progressive conception!

Here are some of the proven natural techniques to manage fainting and stay safe!

- Keep left when you lie down
- When you get up from the bed, first turn to your right side, sit up for some time and gradually put your foot to

the ground and get up

- Ensure your iron level is kept normal as per your report
- Keep yourself hydrated
- Practice yoga and meditation on a daily basis
- Always ensure you are guided by someone if you happened to be traveling to unknown places
- Make sure you have gripped sandals and carpets at home for your safety
- Do not get up abruptly from a sitting or standing position

Headache

You might experience headaches of varying degrees during your pregnancy. It may be due to the massive shift in the blood circulation of the baby.

Headache can be also due to the hormonal effect or because of those sleepless nights you have. Unless it is incapacitating, the following methods would help you calm your head.

- Try to sleep with your legs elevated with a cushion or a soft pillow
- Do not use a pillow while resting your head when you have an episode of headache
- Drink a lot of water to keep yourself full
- Always ensure to eat frequent meals 5 to 6 times
- Lying down on your left side can better your headache and hence this position is better than a sitting or standing position when you have a headache
- Practice relaxation techniques preferably in the early morning or just before you go to bed
- If you work with computers/ LCD screens, take a 3-minute break every 45 minutes of your work

Heartburn

If you do not suffer from any heart diseases, heartburn can be handled lightheartedly and much more effectively!

- Always have small frequent meals rather than going for large options
- Stay away from spicy/ junk foods. If it's quite irresistible, have it minimum
- Keep yourself hydrated and drink less citrous juices if you have severe heartburn and regurgitation
- Include plain salads preferably fresh greens at least for one course of your meals
- Have a piece of dry food like cookies or dried bread as soon as you get up
- Practice yoga and meditation daily

Itching

Your maternal antibodies are more alert during your conception to keep your baby safe. But unfortunately, this process can land up in you developing rashes and itching, and redness during this period. Inadequate hydration can also predispose you to develop itching.

Adopting the following methods can keep your skin healthy!

- Make sure you drink plenty of water and empty your bladder without holding it for a long time
- Practice daily walking for about 15 minutes and do take some shallow fresh air as you move around
- Mix in turmeric and mildly heated coconut oil and apply it to your body for 30 to 45 minutes before bath
- Use natural exfoliants such as green gram powder, Bengal gram powder, or any other natural products to

wash it off
- Use cotton garments as your pregnancy progresses

Mood changes

Mood changes are inevitable in pregnancy, especially for the first time. The recurring symptoms, the ever-growing tummy, backaches, and indigestion surely make your mood swing. That's why I have dedicated several pages of this book explaining the mindfulness and meditation techniques for you and your partner.

Muscle cramps

If you are experiencing pregnancy, there are chances that you will meet with an uninvited muscle cramp, especially during the nighttime. The frequency might increase as you approach your term.

Here are some of the tips that have proven to be beneficial in preventing the cramps (focusing on legs as they are more common):

- Perform regular leg and foot exercises (refer to Chapter 9)
- Do not sit with a twisted leg
- Support your foot whenever possible.
- Do not dangle them, instead raise and support your legs
- Avoid wearing high heels.
- Use flat footwears
- Cover your legs when you sleep.
- Use woolen socks or a good blanket
- Have a weekly oil bath with gentle massages on your whole body, focusing on your legs and foot
- Drink a cup of warm milk at night before you sleep
- Do not use hot applications/ massages if you are taking any blood thinners (medicines like Heparin,

Clopidogrel, etc)

Nausea and Vomiting

Nausea and vomiting can be quite challenging for pregnant women, especially when they consume for the first time. As a health coach, I'm mostly concerned with nausea and vomiting as this issue compromise both the mother's and baby's nutrition. I strongly recommend consulting your healthcare provider and seeking medical help if throwing up incapacitates you to eat or perform your daily activities.

Meanwhile, you can review some of the effective methods to manage nausea and vomiting:

- Have a piece of dried food for 30 minutes to 1 hour before you get up.
- Continue your sleep afterward.
- Eat meals in small but frequent quantities; say 5 to 6 times a day
- Avoid spicy and fast foods
- Keep yourself hydrated by drinking plain water and fresh fruit juice
- Make sure to eat foods with varied tastes rather than going for your regular meals
- Try something different for your taste buds!

Pregnancy Mask

The Pregnancy mask appears in 50 to 70% of pregnant women. The darkening of your skin or dryness or patches appearing on the face might disturb some of the mothers-to-be. But luckily, in most cases, it fades off with your child's birth! Since it is because of the hormonal effect, nothing much can be done to pull off the mask.

However, having a weekly oil bath with turmeric and coconut oil and an occasional face mask with sandal and redwood sandals can render a divine aura on your face!

Regurgitation

You might be familiar with the reasons behind heartburn during pregnancy. Regurgitation also is one of the disturbing symptoms found commonly in pregnant women. Usually, the natural remedies for heartburn work very well for regurgitation too! In addition to those tips, consider the following suggestions as well.

- Support yourself with pillows when you lie down
- Resting for 5 to 10 minutes after your meals, especially after breakfast and dinner either in a sitting or lying down position

Stretch Marks

Just imagine how your skin and muscles in your tummy feel like when they get stretched to thrice or four times their original form! And now you see why the stretch marks are so prominent in your abdomen!

Try the recommended activities for managing stretch marks. These can help you have beautiful and healthy abs after your childbirth!

- Perform pregnancy exercises as early as you can
- Start 3 months before conception Perform regular weekly oil baths with coconut and turmeric oil preferably from your first month onwards
- Apply olive oil or any other natural oil (Ayurvedic) as per the direction of the manufacturers

Swelling of Legs

Like your brain and other organs, the legs too suffer from compromised circulation during pregnancy. The enlarged uterus inhibits the venous return* to the heart and the result is your swollen legs!

Unless you have high blood pressure/ blood sugar, managing your swollen foot is less tiresome. Here are the suggestions:

- Perform leg and foot exercises from your initial stage of pregnancy (refer to Chapter 9)
- Avoid wearing tight footwear or high heels
- Support your legs with a maternity footstool (at the office) or with cushions or pillows when you are at home

Tiredness

Due to the above ailments we discussed, your body will be overloaded with a lot of duties (in addition to your household chores) to look after your baby that, my dear, you will feel tired when you are pregnant!

But once you practice the suggestions given below, you can very well drift smoothly through the journey of pregnancy with more happiness!

- Practice regular yoga and meditation even before you conceive
- Replenish yourself with the right power foods! (refer to A to Z Foods for pregnancy in Appendix - D)
- Hydrate yourself with a good amount of plain water and fresh fruit juices
- Take occasional rest in between your work
- Go out and enjoy your special time by watching or doing your favorite things!

- Play some soothing music before you go to sleep

Urgency or Frequency of Urine

The compressing uterus prompts your bladder to empty too often which creates an urgency for passing urine during pregnancy. The extra fluid from the uterus (the amniotic fluid and the baby's urine) makes an additional amount of urine to be expelled out!

Managing this can be quite disturbing, but unfortunately, this is inevitable as long as this whole process is just meant for your pregnancy to progress in the right way!

However, the following tips can be of your help to get relief from the problems associated with frequent urination.

- Use cotton garments and make sure to change them as and when you get wet
- Do not withhold your urine. Empty your bladder as soon as you can
- Eat citrus fruits throughout the day

CHAPTER NINE

Exercises for Pregnancy

Benefits of performing exercises

- You will get a smart baby!
- Pregnancy becomes a graceful experience
- More chance for Normal Delivery
- Excellent for Baby's mental & Physical growth
- You recover faster after delivery

Pregnancy exercises

1. Breathing exercise
2. Foot and Leg exercise
3. Transversus Abdominis Muscle exercise
4. Pelvic tilting and rocking exercise
5. Pelvic Floor muscle exercise

Breathing Exercises

Benefits

- Helps you increase your self-awareness
- Keeps you calm and comfortable

- Helps you develop acceptance for the body changes you are going through

When to perform?

Start before your pregnancy. However, if you happened to read this book now when you are pregnant, start right away!

Steps

- Sit comfortably with your eyes closed
- Listen to your breathing
- Concentrate on the short pause after the breaths
- Keep your breathing level fairly low down in the chest

How often can you practice breathing exercises?

Several times during the day For up to 2 minutes

Caution Note

- No deep breaths!
- 2 or 3 deep breaths however are safe for you and your baby!

Leg and Foot Exercises

Benefits

Prevents:

- Edema or swelling
- Leg cramps
- Leg pain
- Improves circulation

Steps

- Sit comfortably Bend and stretch the ankles at least 12 times
- Circle both feet at the ankle at least 20 times in clockwise and anti-clockwise directions
- Now brace both your knees, holding for a count of four
- Once you are done, relax and bring back your knees to the normal position
- Repeat 12 times

Tips:

- Avoid prolonged standing
- Do not sit cross-legged
- Go flat with footwear
- Elevate your feet whenever seated

Transverse Abdominis Muscle (TVA)Exercises
How to perform (TVA) Exercises?
Steps
You may perform this exercise sitting or standing. In the early stages of pregnancy, you can perform kneeling on all fours as well.

- Sit comfortably
- Pull in the lower part of the abdomen below the umbilicus
- Keep your spine still
- Hold up for up to 10 seconds
- Relax
- Repeat 10 times

When to perform?

Whenever you stand or while doing any activities Also, when you handle heavy object

Pelvic Muscle Exercise

Benefits

- Minimize pressure on your back, Urinary bladder, and Joints
- Prevent aching legs
- Relieve breathing difficulty
- Alleviate indigestion
- Equip your body to provide good support for your baby
- Brighten the pregnancy period

Pelvic Tilt

When to perform pelvic tilts?

Whenever you stand For better results, master this exercise before pregnancy

Pelvic Tilt in detail:

Steps to perform pelvic tilt:

Head

Do's

Lift through the crown of the head and keep your chin lifted in line with your neck

Dont's

Chin pulling forwards and eyes focused down

Shoulder

Do's

Draw your shoulders back and down while you lift the rib cage up

Dont's

Slouching your shoulders and rib cage. (This makes your breathing more difficult and put you at risk of developing indigestion)

Abdomen, Buttocks, and Uterus

Do's

Contract abdominals to support your baby Tuck your butt under and tilt the pubis or pelvic bone slightly forward to the center of the pelvic bowl

Dont's

Letting your tummy jut out! (Weak muscles allow out the back and tilt your pelvis forward causing backache, strained abdominals, and excess pressure on your bladder)

Feet

Do's

Spread your feet or leave an ideal gap between your feet while standing. Distribute your body weight over the center of each foot

Dont's

Attempting to support your body weight with a single leg or trying to distribute your body weight to the inner aspect of your feet will strain your calves causing leg pain

Knees

Do's

Bend knees to ease body weight over feet

Dont's

Pressing your knees backward (This will cause pain in your joints and eventually tilt your pelvis which is undesirable)

Exercise for Rectus Abdominus Muscle

Benefits

- Tone up the muscles of the back and pelvis
- Helps you experience more comfort during your labor
- Prevents lifelong back ailments
- Strengthen ligaments thereby protecting you from complications

- Helps tone up your abdomen

Steps

- You can perform this exercise in a half-lying position, raising your upper body with a pillow
- Bend your knees and keep your feet flat
- Place one hand under the small of your back and the other on the top of the abdomen
- Tighten the abdominals and buttocks, and press the small of the back down on the underneath hand
- Hold for up to 10 seconds then relax
- Repeat 10 times

Pelvic Floor Muscle Exercises

Benefits

- Provides good support to the uterus
- Helps you to 'push' effectively during labor
- Prevents later complications of labor such as leakage of urine while coughing

Steps

- Sit, stand, or half-lie with legs slightly apart
- Close and draw up as though preventing a bowel action
- Simultaneously, close and draw up around the front passage as though preventing urination
- Draw up inside and hold up for as long as possible, up to 10 seconds
- You can also perform this exercise by stopping your midstream while urinating and immediately releasing the urine

- Relax and repeat up to 10 times

CHAPTER TEN

Sexuality and Pregnancy

A period of separation for couples?

A handful of factors prevent intimacy between the partners during pregnancy. The possible reasons for a couple to not have intercourse would be tiredness or emotional unreadiness that might be due to the mother's hormonal changes. In some cases, the parents-to-be are simply worried if it would cause damage to their baby. In India, several cultures also restrain the couple from having an intimate relationship during pregnancy.

Dealing with Facts

While several kinds of research support there is no harm in having intercourse during pregnancy, one may need to consider several facts while dealing with the childbearing phase.

Supporting and understanding your female partner would ease things and lead to more emotional and physical intimacy during pregnancy. Feel free to talk out your thoughts and explore what's in her head too! Spend a good amount of time together to discuss how you can address the safety concern while having sex. Your treating doctor may be of great help when you have questions about your medical conditions and their effect on your sexuality.

Caution if you have these conditions:

You are advised to have intercourse with utmost caution if you have the following conditions:

- Vaginal bleeding
- Fungal infection
- Placenta previa - You have the Placenta placed downwards (abnormal position)
- Premature dilatation of the cervix - Your Doctor has mentioned that you have this condition during your visit
- Rupture of the membranes - You have broken your water well early on your expected delivery date in the past
- History of premature delivery - You have delivered before reaching the term of pregnancy in the past (before 9 months)
- Multiple pregnancies - You are carrying more than one child in your tummy

It is essential that you understand and connect with each other for maintaining love and intimacy during pregnancy. You may carry on with the simple act of caring and sharing with the mother-to-be and enjoy your special moments of togetherness.

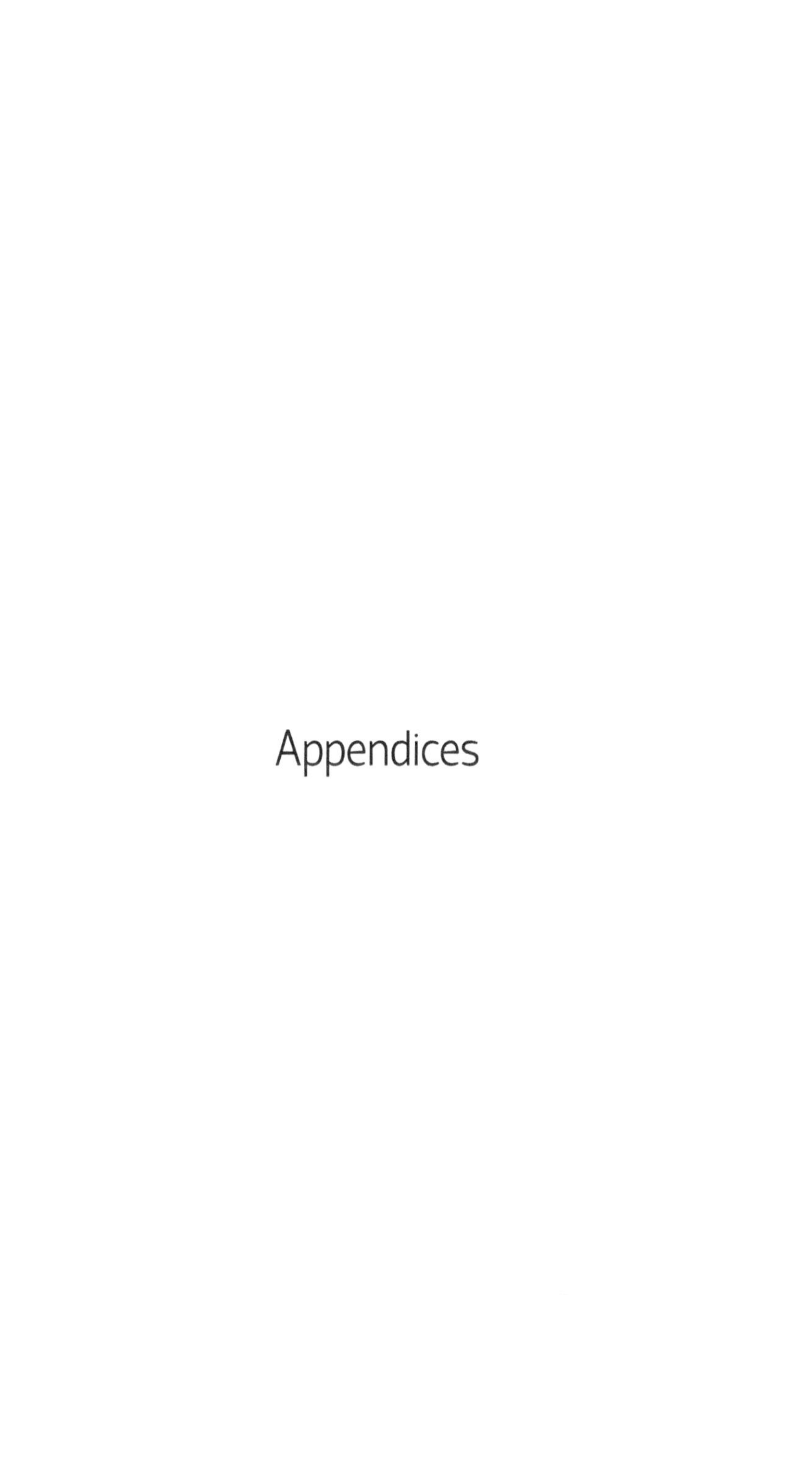

Appendices

Appendix – A Terminology

Meaning of some of the vocabularies you might be interested in looking into!

Embryo

In humans, an embryo is a developing organism from the fourth day after fertilization to the end of the eighth week.

Fetal Macrosomia

In a newborn, birth weight above 4000 grams.

APGAR Score

A score (method) for determining an infant's condition at birth by scoring the heart rate, respiratory effort, muscle tone, reflex irritability, and color. The infant is rated from 0 to 2 on each of the five items, the highest possible score being 10

Neural Tube Defect

A congenital defect in the closure of the bony encasement of the spinal cord or of the skull. The most severe defects are a fissure along the entire length of the spinal column that leaves the meninges and spinal cord exposed, or herniation through the skull of a saclike structure containing brain tissue and meninges

Fetus

In humans, the product of conception is from the end of the eighth week to the moment of birth.

BMI (Body Mass Index)

Body Mass Index is a simple calculation using a person's height and weight. The formula is BMI = kg/m2 where kg is a person's weight in kilograms and m2 is their height in meters squared. A BMI of 25.0 or more is overweight, while the healthy range is 18.5 to 24.9. During pregnancy and lactation, a woman's body composition changes, so using BMI is not appropriate.

Conception/Fertilisation

The fusion of male and female gametes to produce a new organism.

Umbilical cord

The long flexible tubelike structure connecting a fetus with the placenta: it provides a means of metabolic interchange with the mother.

Vernix caseosa

A white cheese-like protective material that covers the skin of a fetus.

Lanugo

A covering of fine, soft hair, especially that found on the unborn baby or newborn.

Umbilicus

Synonym of the navel.

Xiphisternum

the cartilaginous process forming the lowermost part of the breastbone (sternum).

Musculoskeletal

Related to the muscles and bones.

Palpation

To examine or explore by touching (an organ or area of the body), usually as a diagnostic aid.

Diaphragm

A muscular membranous partition separating the abdominal and thoracic cavities and functioning in respiration

Pica

A psychiatric disorder is characterized by the compulsive eating of nonfood substances, such as soil, clay, ice, or hair.

Gastroesophageal sphincter

A ring of smooth muscle fibers at the junction of the esophagus and stomach.

Preeclampsia

A condition of hypertension occurring in pregnancy is typically accompanied by swelling and the presence of protein in the urine. Also called toxemia of pregnancy.

Gestational Diabetes Mellitus

A disorder characterized by an impaired ability to metabolize carbohydrates, usually caused by a deficiency of insulin or insulin resistance, occurs in pregnancy. It disappears after delivery of the infant but, in a significant number of cases, returns years later as type 2 diabetes mellitus

Appendix – B Tips For The Daddies – To – Be

Home and surroundings

1. Go for a spring clean when you start your pregnancy plan. It will help you both feel calm and content.

2. Ensure the mommy seldom gets to breathe the fresh paint when you prepare your home to welcome your young one.

3. Make sure the slippery floors are laid down with carpets for your lady to walk smoothly and safely.

4. Ensure a thorough cleaning through vacuuming every weekend.

Dealing with Emotional dilemma

1. Cope up with her mood changes and help her accept the possible changes during pregnancy.

2. Taking her on small walks will ease her body and mind in addition to bringing both of you even closer.

3. You don't have to change the entire you to be a 'Dad', but do express your love to her so often that she and your growing young one will feel secure.

4. Join her during her meditation and prayer sessions. Trust me, this will bring more miracles in your family life. 5. Ensure your well-being too with adequate sleep and hangouts with your friends. Being too alert will soon drain your energy level. Keep calm and enjoy your part in bringing your younger ones as you offer your help to your partner.

Food

1. Do not try to include new food during the pregnancy period.

2. Make sure you buy no preserved or old foods for her.

3. Keep an eye on her sugar intake, especially when your partner is having gestational diabetes. Women can have cravings during pregnancy which is quite natural but ensure she takes foods that are allowed during pregnancy.

4. Clean up your fridge and substitute beverages and fruit cans with fruits.

5. Encourage her to eat a lot of locally available fruits and vegetables. They can be an excellent source of nutrients for your baby. It won't burn your pocket too!

6. Always make sure to fill the containers on your dining table with water and fresh fruits. By doing so, she might not feel forced into focusing on a lot of foods all the time.

Workouts

1. I highly recommend you work out together. This will ensure her safety and it's always fun to perform exercises with your partner!

2. Talk to your health care provider about the exercise, if there is any modification, etc as and when the pregnancy progresses.

3. An excellent suggestion is going for walks in the morning. Practice this golden tip when you plan for your pregnancy.

Body Care

1. Support her as she goes through the inevitable transformation stages of pregnancy. Reassure her that it is normal and don't forget to express your love is intact no matter how she looks

2. Give her an oil bath with gentle massages. This will take your intimacy and trust to another level

3. She might suffer from skin irritations; make sure you help her apply moisturizer, especially during the nighttime.

4. Be careful while giving leg massages or giving hot compress if your partner is receiving any class of Anticoagulant medications such as Warfarin or Heparin during pregnancy. Talk to your provider for the right method.

5. Buy her pregnancy-supporting pillows as pregnancy progresses. Ensure she is lying on her left.

6. Ensure nothing constricts her tummy, such as a tight-fitting cloth or your car's seat belt.

Appendix – C Did You Know?

Babies can taste the food!

Did you know that your baby can taste the food you eat in a period as early as when you are 3 months pregnant? What's more, your pregnancy nutrition can be more likely to shape your baby's food preference in its later life! So no more thoughts, eat right and give your baby delicious delight of the variant food delicacies each day!

Memory Loss during Pregnancy or Momnesia

During your pregnancy, you are more likely to forget things that can make you feel weird! Yes, memory loss or 'Amnesia' or even called 'Momnesia' literally is characterized by forgetfulness ranging from variant degrees. You can manage this condition very effectively with a couple of techniques on your own!

Beware of the vessels you use for cooking!

Did you know that you are prone to ingest chemicals present in the cooking vessels that might pose risk to both the mother and baby? Choosing the right cooking vessels keeps you safe during pregnancy.

Vacuuming and Pregnancy

Did you know that performing household chores such as mopping and vacuuming can make your back and legs ache? Your incorrect posture during pregnancy can pave the way to such issues which can be very well prevented if you practice good postures during pregnancy!

Your voice calms your baby!

By the seventh or eighth month, your baby's sensory system is so well developed that it can listen to various sounds from your burps to the sounds in your surroundings! The fascinating fact is that, among these sounds, it is the mother's voice that the baby familiarizes with. Your baby's heartbeat slows down each time it hears your voice, indicating that it has a soothing effect!

More Vitamin A, but do you really need it?

An overdosage of Vitamin A even when you're 1 month pregnant can put your baby at risk of developing several vision defects. All you have to do to stay safe is to go for simple dietary tips which you will find in our course

Want an emotionally and physically healthy baby? Go Meditation mode!

Your baby's nervous system develops at an early stage (before you are even aware that you are pregnant)! You don't have to take extra effort to have a wise baby! All you have to do is to sit in your room quietly and meditate! There are several mindfulness and meditation videos available on the internet.

If you are a beginner, you may begin with a one-minute meditation slowly progressing to a longer duration. You may also indulge in visiting religious or sacred places as per your cultural norms.

Appendix – D A To Z Foods For Your Pregnancy

Apple

Embrace this fruit during your pregnancy because this superfood has the proven power to safeguard you from developing gestational diabetes, preeclampsia, heart disease, constipation, swollen feet, and several infections that can be detrimental to the fetus during pregnancy.

The benefit to the fetus includes the protection this food offers you from the poisonous substance that may enter your body during the conception period. Apple also prevents the breakdown of DNA thereby reducing the chances of birth defects in your baby. Several kinds of research show that consuming apples can save your baby from developing asthma and other respiratory disorders later in its life.

Caution

Talk with your healthcare provider about your intake limit if you suffer from diabetes.

Tip

Eat an apple on your empty stomach.

Beans

Beans include a variety of white, black, green, and French ones. The brimming vitamins and amino acids in addition to several microelements make this wonder food 'vegetarian meat'! Consuming beans from an early period of pregnancy will improve your fertility. Eating beans from the period of your family planning will also supply your body with adequate iron. As you know iron is the major component in the production of hemoglobin, it will thus give you a good blood count during pregnancy. It will also help you from developing high blood pressure and issues related to malnutrition (especially with the proteins if you are a vegetarian).

Niacin present in beans will help your baby's nervous growth development, not to mention those wonderful nails and hair your baby would be getting! In addition to this, the protein present in the bean (which is almost equivalent to meat), will help in the proper growth and development of your baby during pregnancy.

Tips

- Include bean dishes in your daily diet. Soak in the beans (locally available) overnight
- Grind it in the morning
- Mix the paste with a teaspoon of olive oil and lemon juice
- Apply it all over your body and leave for 15 to 20 minutes
- Wash it off to see a younger and divine body!

Berries and Fruits

These superfoods are indispensable during your pregnancy and even before it! Eating fruits daily from 3 to 6 months of your family planning will give you a safe and healthy pregnancy. The nutrients present in fruits will reduce the risk of various diseases such as diabetes, blood pressure, constipation, and heart disorders.

Fruits and berries will provide an excellent environment to excel in its growth and development. They protect your baby from birth defects and genetic disorders, especially in case of late pregnancy.

Tips

- Smash up some berries and fruits to savor smoothies

during the daytime
- Apply mashed fruits, especially grapes and berries as a face mask throughout your pregnancy

Carrot

Consuming carrots during pregnancy can have innumerable benefits for you and your baby. Chewing raw carrots can soothe your swollen gums during pregnancy and acts as a toothbrush to cleanse your teeth and gums. They also help sustain a steady sugar level in your bloodstream keeping you energetic and light all through the day!

Tips

- Enjoy juices and halwas during your weekends!
- Crunch in some fresh carrots in the morning preferably during your preconception period and first trimester of pregnancy

Coconut

Coconut could be consumed in its fresh form or as coconut oil. You can also drink fresh coconut water, or fresh coconut sprouts from your pregnancy till the breastfeeding period. This nutrient-enriched food will help your body replenish with essential components such as vitamins, minerals, and essential electrolytes such as sodium and potassium. Coconut will enable you to feel full while providing your digestive system with ease to work on!

Having coconut during your pregnancy will keep you energized, rescue you from morning sickness, and protects you from several infections.

Your baby will have excellent nervous system development. The coconut should be on your 'must list' if you long for a baby with a good head, heart, and hair!

Caution

- Do not consume coconut if it's exposed for more than 3 hours in the open air
- Also, avoid processed coconut (that comes in tin) in the first trimester of your pregnancy

Tips

- Cook simple coconut chutneys once or twice a week.
- Use grated coconut for the boiled pulses for your evening snacks Consume tender coconut water for morning sickness/ vomiting during pregnancy
- Apply coconut milk all over your body (including your head) for 15 to 20 minutes once a week and wash it off with a natural exfoliant

Dark Chocolate

Good news for all those 'mommies to be' chocolate lovers! Research has proved that eating chocolates can keep your head and heart, healthy in addition to giving you good moods! It can also prevent preeclampsia and other heart diseases during pregnancy.

Consuming this food will have enhanced benefits on your baby's Intelligent Quotient (IQ) and Emotional Quotient (EI). Consuming chocolates can protect your baby from several diseases because of the antioxidants present in them.

Caution

- Talk to your health care provider regarding your limit if you have diabetes.
- Eat in moderation. Overeating can lead to obesity and hence can affect your fertility and pregnancy

Tips

- Have a piece of chocolate with a glass of milk before you sleep
- Having a bite of dark chocolates during the morning will supply you with a good mood throughout the day

Egg

This superfood is rich in components for cell growth and repair, and hence it is the best-recommended food during pregnancy! Eating an egg right from your preconception period, say, three months will supply your body with adequate calcium, proteins, and other vital elements. Your baby will benefit from getting excellent nervous development, weight gain, and musculoskeletal development. Eating eggs in your early trimester will safeguard your baby from birth defects and developmental delays.

Tips

- Include egg with pepper for your breakfast
- Apply egg white with lemon juice on your face and neck
- Leave for 20 minutes and wash it off

Caution

- Do not consume raw eggs
- See the carton for the details of the date of packing

- Avoid eating old-stock eggs

Fish

Fishes are the cheapest source of nutrients during your pregnancy. Eating fishes like tuna and sardines are good sources of Omega 3 fatty acids and DHA, the vital components for your baby's brain and its associated growth and development. Since the neural tube (primitive nervous system) is formed as early as four weeks of pregnancy (even before you realize you are pregnant), consuming fish during your preconception period will save your baby from developmental delays.

Fishes are an excellent source of vitamins, proteins, calcium, and essential electrolytes. Hence including fish in your daily diet during pregnancy will fill your body with all the extra nutrients it needs for this period. The good cholesterol (HDL) present in the fish will keep a check on your weight gain and of course, give you a healthy heart!

Caution

- Take care when you buy tuna as it can contain excess mercury that is detrimental to the fetus
- Consume very less tuna and sushi during your first trimester

Tips

- Include stewed fish with pepper for your lunch
- Consume more freshwater fish prepared with coconut milk

Ghee

Ghee is a wonderful food that can improve your cognition and mood during pregnancy. Consuming pure ghee during your pregnancy will enhance your baby's neural development and have an excellent result on its intellectual abilities in later life! Having ghee before three months of your pregnancy will prove beneficial not only to the baby but also to your digestive system!

Ghee provides essential nutrients such as calcium, vitamins, and other components during your conception period. It smoothens your gut, thereby preventing constipation and hemorrhoids associated with decreased intestinal motility (during pregnancy).

Tips

- Have a teaspoon of ghee in the early morning
- Try Indian Desserts or Banana fry with grated coconuts using ghee as the cooking oil in mild to moderate amounts

Himalayan Salt

Himalayan salt is the best alternative for the 'vegan mommies' as the sulfur present in this powerful salt is equivalent to that in the egg yolk. Substitute this salt for your table salt and give your baby a good head and hair!

Tip

Use Himalayan salt for your swollen feet and leg pain.

Honey

Honey has several medicinal properties and hence it was recommended for pregnant women in the ancient Indian scriptures written several thousands of years ago. They all suggest the use of honey during pregnancy for getting a child with higher intelligence.

Consuming honey has several other benefits for the expecting mother too. It enhances your metabolism, cognition, and mood.

Using honey for treating skin ailments is also recommended during this period. This is because of its healing properties and no side effects compared to modern medicines.

Tips

- Have a tablespoon of honey with $1/4^{th}$ of lemon juice in the early morning
- Substitute honey for white sugar

Caution

Ensure the honey you consume is pasteurized.

Jaggery

Jaggery has surplus benefits and hence it is highly recommended during your pregnancy as well as breastfeeding period. The rich antioxidants present in jaggery will remove all your impurities in addition to boosting your immune power. The rich content of iron will meet your extra requirement for the formation of hemoglobin too. Jaggery has certain medicinal properties too. So it is wise to substitute for sugar.

Caution

Talk to your health care provider about the limit if you suffer from diabetes.

Tip

- Use palm jaggery (liquid or solidified) as it is superior in medicinal properties
- Prepare desserts aka kheer or payasam with jaggery on weekends

Kale/Spinach

Spinach is the best form of folic acid among the food readily available. Hence it is highly recommended to include them in your daily diet. Both partners can consider a wide range of spinach/kale preparation. It is best if you can include all the colored varieties of this leafy wonder. Your baby can get benefited from its rich nutrients such as Vitamin A, D, C, and K, Vitamin B12, B6, iron, calcium, and magnesium. The results are better neural development of your baby in addition to the proper development of its vision, bones, and muscles.

Caution

- Ensure proper washing and check thoroughly when you prepare fresh salads
- Talk with your health care provider if you are on any anti-coagulants as the intake of green leafy vegetables may interfere with the action of the medicine

Tip

Prepare spinach dishes with the combination of pulses such as dal, tubers such as potato, grated coconut, or any other foods that goes great along with this superfood.

Lemon

The brimming Vitamin C in lemon will give you the essential platform for skin repair and growth. Drinking lemonades during pregnancy will help rejuvenate the body cells and thus enables you and your baby to have healthy skins. It will also keep you refreshed and aids in preventing nausea. Lemon increases the palatability of food during pregnancy.

The antioxidants present in this fruit will destroy free radicals in your body safeguarding the baby inside your womb. It will improve both the mother's and the baby's immunity as well.

Caution

- Restrict the use of lemon if you suffer from acidity/ regurgitation
- Stop the intake of lemon if you develop a dislike or if consuming it aggravates your vomiting or constipation, you can discontinue its use

Tips

- Squeeze fresh lemon juice into your salads, sprouts, fish, and meat dishes
- Add mint to lemonade to enhance its flavor and palatability
- Add lemon juice to the freshly prepared juices

Meat

Meat is an inevitable one in the food family that can supply you with major proteins required for the building and repair of your body cells during pregnancy. Consuming meat can give you enough proteins, iron, calcium, magnesium, and other vitamins and minerals that can meet increased demand as your pregnancy progresses.

Consuming meat will supply your baby with enough nutrients for its overall growth and development, especially, that of its muscles and bones.

Caution

- Avoid liver and liver products during pregnancy
- Avoid raw/ old/ tinned/ processed meat
- Do not consume undercooked/ burnt/ charred meat

Tips

Prefer stews rather than deep-fries for meat dishes Consume fresh green salads along with the meat course

Milk and Milk products

Milk has almost all essential nutrients required for your pregnancy and no wonder with its composition of these elements, it is referred to as the complete food. Both the partners can include milk and its products in their daily diet as early as 3 to six months before pregnancy. But when the mother is pregnant, increase her milk intake further. Ensure it is derived from a healthy source (For example - Antibiotic-free milk or a freshly delivered milk if you have such access.

Drinking milk during pregnancy has a positive effect on the birth weight of your baby and could contribute to better health in its later life too. Consuming milk and milk products can supply your baby with adequate calcium and magnesium required for its musculoskeletal development.

Caution

- Do not drink raw milk and raw cheeses, especially during the first trimester of your pregnancy
- Ensure you are getting high-quality milk or 'Desi' milk to consume

Tips

- Cook a wide variety of dishes with milk so that you won't feel drinking milk is a chore
- Prepare sweet dishes with milk and milk solids
- Consume goat milk in the early morning

Oils

You can use a variety of oils such as olive oil, coconut oil, fish oil, mustard oil, and several other edible oils depending on your geographical location and cultural practice. However, the first three oils can replenish your body with their unique nutrients that will benefit you and your baby throughout the pregnancy period. Consuming oils (in moderation) can help in relieving some of your pregnancy symptoms. They provide you with good fat and hence their benefits are proven for your cardiovascular system (heart and blood vessels).

Consuming coconut oil can improve your baby's cognition and other intelligent functions while olive oil will fight against all those stressful free radicals in your body. Fish oils provide an excellent source of micro and macro elements needed by your growing baby in addition to the Omega 3 fatty acids and DHA.

Caution

- Please refer to your healthcare provider for your limit on consuming oils if you have any diseases
- Do not heat virgin oils instead sprinkle them in your freshly prepared salads
- Do not reheat the used oils

Tips

- Prepare coconut oil at home or get it from places that prepare them on a small scale
- Consume a teaspoon of coconut oil on empty stomach to relieve the symptom of constipation

Orange

Oranges are the most reliable source of energy for your vitamin C requirement. It is also a storehouse of calcium and folic acid which are crucial for the initial stages of your pregnancy. Oranges can relieve your morning sickness/ vomiting during pregnancy too.

Consuming oranges can give a divine glow to your baby in addition to those healthy brains and muscles, but make sure both the partners include oranges or any citrus fruits in your daily diet from the period of your pregnancy planning.

Caution

- Limit the intake of citrus fruits/ oranges if you suffer from any acidity/ gastric issues
- Do not heat these food groups as you will immediately lose the nutrients as soon as it contacts the heat

Tips

- Prefer eating the whole orange to the juice as the former can supply you with more fiber
- Apply orange juice onto your face regularly for 5 to 10 minutes and wash them off with plain water to give yourself a golden glow

Quinoa

Quinoa is the best choice for expectant mothers who suffer from gluten sensitivity. This food is your best choice if you are a vegan mommy-to-be! Quinoa is one of the rare plants which has all the essential amino acids (normally we rely on red meat, chicken, and eggs for the same). Eating quinoa during pregnancy can be a healthy option to have a check on your body weight too!

Now, for your baby, this wonder food will supply the tiny one with an excellent volume of vitamin B, and folic acid which is very important during its initial growth.

Caution

Ensure thorough washing of the seeds as their coating can be irritant to your stomach.

Tip

Include more quinoa dishes if you are diabetic.

Rice

From managing your bowel movements to delaying aging; unpolished rice has several benefits. Rice when taken in the porridge form can provide sustained release of sugar to your bloodstream giving you a steady pace of energy level throughout the day.

Your baby can have wholesome benefits from rice. It can have improved muscle and skin development during the intrauterine period, and have a comparatively healthy birth weight when born. Rice can also help improve intellectual abilities in its later life.

Caution

- Limit the intake of polished rice, instead, consume the unpolished one
- Talk to your healthcare provider about your carbohydrate limit if you suffer from diabetes

Tips

- Have rice porridge with freshly prepared chutneys of your choice for dinner. This will aid in bowel movement and reduction of constipation and digestion issues
- Apply rice powder with milk and tomato juice mixed well onto your face and neck. Leave for 20 to 30

minutes. Wash it off to have a younger skin!

Seafood

Seafood is best recommended even from the initial stage of your family planning because of its positive effect on fertility. They are the storehouse of zinc, omega 3 fatty acid, DHA, and other microelements that are proven to boost your reproductive function.

For your baby, the nutrients present in various kinds of seafood will prevent birth defects or other anomalies. These superfoods will also aid in your baby's intellectual abilities.

Caution

Watch for mercury poisoning when you consume seafood Ensure you consume them well cooked.

Tips

Sprinkle lemon juice or eat citrous fruit to enhance the seafood's absorption.

Turmeric

Turmeric is best known for its divine properties to cleanse your body. If you follow the Indian diet, there is no need to include turmeric as extra. However, this ingredient will always be of your help if you encounter any infections during your pregnancy. Your baby eventually gets benefited from the antioxidant properties of turmeric.

Caution

Avoid over usage of turmeric as it can lead to toxicity.

Tip

Boil milk with a pinch of turmeric added to it to relieve your lung congestion. Drink it before going to bed. Grind fresh turmeric root and mix it with sandal paste. Apply it all over your body and leave it for 1 hour. Wash it off with a natural exfoliant. Repeat at least once a month during your pregnancy.

Turmeric

Turmeric is best known for its divine properties to cleanse your body. If you follow the Indian diet, there is no need to include turmeric as extra. However, this ingredient will always be of your help if you encounter any infections during your pregnancy. Your baby eventually gets benefited from the antioxidant properties of turmeric.

Caution

Avoid over usage of turmeric as it can lead to toxicity.

Tip

- Boil milk with a pinch of turmeric added to it to relieve your lung congestion
- Drink it before going to bed
- Grind fresh turmeric root and mix it with sandal paste
- Apply it all over your body and leave it for 1 hour.
- Wash it off with a natural exfoliant. Repeat at least once a month during your pregnancy

Unsalted Nuts

Unsalted nuts are the best way to find good cholesterol and stay in shape during your pregnancy. They also contain plenty of nutrients to keep your mind and body full of enthusiasm. Eating nuts during pregnancy can supply your baby with essential nutrients for its growth and development.

Caution

Do not consume any new nuts during pregnancy. Beware of nut allergy.

Tip

- Crumble the nuts and sprinkle them in your salads and

breakfast, rather than consuming them as a whole
- Drink milk or yogurt along if you are taking a comparatively large amount of nuts

Vegetables

I cannot mention each vegetable and hence I have mentioned some of the significant ones for your pregnancy in the 'A to Z foods'. By vegetables, I mean to suggest to you the colorful varieties. Vegetables are the storehouses of vitamins and a whole lot of energies they derive directly from the sun (unlike meat and egg products). Hence including them in your meals will suffice your energy requirement for a normal being.

The vitamins, minerals, and micro and macronutrients present in vegetables will nourish your baby to develop into a healthy individual with a good emotional, intelligent, and spiritual quotient in the future!

Caution

- Wash the vegetables thoroughly
- Put them in turmeric water overnight if possible to nullify the effect of pesticides present in them
- Do not try any new variety of vegetables during your pregnancy, especially during the first trimester

Tips

- Start growing herbs and spinach in your vegetable garden during your family planning period
- The fresher you consume them, the better. Include at least four different colors of vegetables for your meals per week
- Consuming cucumber, onion, lettuce, cauliflower, etc

does not add up your weight, and hence eat them as much as you can!

Wheat

Wheat is one of the ancient food in our history. Including wheat in your daily diet will provide you with enough energy to go on for the day. Wheat help build muscles as well. It is the best choice if you have diabetes. It also helps you lose excess weight. So it is always a win-win food! Your baby will similarly benefit from the nutrients present in wheat. They will give your young one strong bones and muscles and of course good head and skin too!

Caution

- Beware of gluten allergy.
- Ensure you cook wheat properly before eating

Xigua aka Watermelon

Watermelon is the best choice for your hydration throughout the pregnancy trimesters. Its amazing properties would make your days feel lighter. Since the fruit has more water content, it satiates your thirst and hunger at the same time.

Tips

- Enjoy watermelons preferably during the day rather than in the evening
- Avoid adding sugar to it
- You can savor the fruit cut into small pieces

Yogurt

Yogurt is another wonderful superfood for your pregnancy, especially if you are a vegan mom! Since yogurt contains a good amount of protein, it can meet some of the requirements of protein during pregnancy. Since yogurt is derived from milk, it contains almost the same nutrients in it. It has excellent benefits on your bowel movements as it prevents constipation and digestion issues especially when you enter your second trimester.

Caution

- Beware of gluten allergy
- Ensure you cook wheat properly before eating

Zucchini

Finally Zucchini! Though it looks similar to the Cucumber, both belong to a different families. Consuming zucchini would replenish your body with loads of vitamins and fiber. It eases your digestive issues during your pregnancy. This wonder vegetable would help in emptying your bowel making you feel more comfortable towards your last trimester of pregnancy.

Tips

- You can cook zucchini as per the method adopted in your culture
- Since it does not build up calories, fill them plenty in your salad plate

Appendix - E Faqs

What are the types of deliveries in pregnancy?

*Childbirth can be through natural methods, Caesarean section, and assisted ones. Let's look into each in detail.

1. Natural birth

The baby moves down through the vagina and is expelled from the uterus by the force exerted by the powerful muscle contractions in the uterus, and is assisted by contractions of the muscles in the wall of the abdomen and the diaphragm as the mother voluntarily pushes.

2. Caesarean Section

A spinal or epidural anesthetic is given to the mother, and the baby is usually delivered within five minutes. After delivery, the longer and more complex task of repairing the womb and abdominal muscles is undertaken. In most cases, the scar of a cesarean is low and horizontal, below the bikini line, to avoid any disfigurement.

3. Assisted Labour

Different methods include Artificial Rupture of Membrane (ARM), Forceps and Vacuum delivery, and the use of drugs to induce labor. These are used to ensure maternal and child safety when the natural birth gets interrupted due to various reasons.

Content adapted from Dr. Warwick Carter's Pregnancy A to Z.

What are the normal levels of LDH (Cholesterol) during 3rd trimester of pregnancy?

LDH levels rise during the pregnancy due to various reasons hence it is difficult to give an accurate answer.

However, in general, it depends on maternal well-being. To meet the increasing demand of the growing baby, the fat metabolism or breakdown of fat molecules is at a much faster pace during pregnancy. Hence it is not abnormal if high values of LDH are present in your blood result.

These components are released when tissue damage occurs and there are chances women with high blood pressure and other endocrine disorder (like Thyroid) may present with a high LDH in their blood test.

It is always safe to co-relate your result with your Health Care Providers as they know your medical history better than we do.

What is the benefit of walking during pregnancy?

Walking is beneficial all through the nine months!

For a woman with no other disease, a daily walk of 15 minutes in the Morning Sun can be helpful. Walking also aids in having a natural birth (it helps in bringing the baby downwards) as you near your labor.

Please seek advice from your obstetrician regarding your level of activity if you have:

a. the Previous history of miscarriage, bleeding, complicated delivery

b. You presently suffer from conditions such as gestational diabetes, high blood pressure, or any other abnormality

5 Foods to consider during pregnancy if you're underweight!

Foods form an excellent platform for you and your baby to meet your holistic health during pregnancy. Apart from the nutrient it supplies, food is an excellent conductor of good vibes in your body too! These five food suggestions are the best if you are underweight during your conception period. Ladies who plan their pregnancy can also give it a try!

1. Cereals and whole grains

No other foods than the cereal family will supply you with rich carbs and hence calories required for you during your pregnancy. Make sure you consume them as a whole rather than going for the processed one as the latter loses most of the nutrients during its processing. Opting for fortified cereals can also be a good idea for a kick-start morning!

2. Milk with Ghee

From the ancient Indian texts to modern research, Milk and ghee are considered divine because of the benefits they provide for both your baby and you!

Consuming fresh milk with ghee in the morning will not only fulfill the calorie requirement for a day to start with, but it will sharpen the intellectual wiring of your young one growing inside your tummy as well!

3. Meat

If you are underweight and have a low hemoglobin count (Anemia), meat is the best reliable food. They contain a high amount of protein, various minerals such as Iron, Calcium, Magnesium, Zinc, Potassium, and vitamins such as Vitamin A, C, B-12, and B -6 all of which are crucial for your baby's growth and development. I'm sure you might be well informed not to consume liver or liver products during your pregnancy.

4. Eggs

When you're underweight, your natural fighting mechanism fades because your body itself is fighting to stand up on its own! Don't worry, we have eggs with nutrient-laden components!

Consuming an egg, especially for your breakfast will energize you to carry out your daily chores with more ease. Eating eggs during your third trimester will have a significant effect on the weight gain of your baby too. Pregnant women are however advised to stay away from raw eggs due to the chance of infection and hence the danger it poses for their tiny ones.

5. Banana

In addition to replenishing your body with vitamins, minerals, and protein, it contains high levels of tryptophan which gets converted into serotonin, the 'happiness hormone'!In addition to replenishing your body with vitamins, minerals, and protein, it contains high levels of tryptophan which gets converted into serotonin, the 'happiness hormone'!

Consult your physician and dietician for the portion of banana allowed if you have any restrictions on sugar intake if you are diagnosed with Diabetes or Gestational Diabetes

If a husband and wife have the same blood group (B+), will there be any problems conceiving a baby?

No, there won't be. You will have issues only if you have an Rh-negative factor or in simple terms, a negative blood group, and you're impregnated with a man with a positive (Rh+) blood group.

If the baby growing inside your womb is having Rh-positive factor (or a positive blood group), such blood will be considered a foreign body. As a part of the mother's defense mechanism, the maternal body starts destructing the fetal blood cells.

But do not worry! The condition will be taken care of by your Doctor by administering you the doses of medicines (Rh shots) during the pregnancy.

Meditation for a happy baby!

Meditation is the bliss tonic for a Soul searching for serenity! And when it's done during your pregnancy, it's a win-win situation for both the mommy and the baby!

Here is a powerful meditation technique 'Breathing exercise with your baby in mind' that would have a positive effect on your pregnancy such as :

- Stabilizing your mood as the pregnancy advances
- Enhancing the fetal well-being by having a positive effect on its neural wiring
- Making your baby emotionally stable during its later adulthood
- Ready to learn the how-to meditate?? Here we are, mommy!

Breathing exercise with your baby in mind

- Sit in an open space preferably in a park or on the greens
- Close your eyes and take one to two deep breaths
- Place both your hands on your tummy and imagine you're holding your baby gently with those hands
- Give your baby your lovely smile (if you are shy, you can place an imaginary smile on your face!)
- Now focus on your breath; the normal breaths that you take in.
- Concentrate on the feeling of air entering through your nostril, and its path, and imagine it entering your lungs
- Imagine that air you just took is being delivered to your baby for its growth. Your baby is taking each breath that you are taking!
- Breath out the air as if you are giving out all the unwanted thoughts, feelings, and things you consider isn't good for you
- Sit calm and continue taking 15 to 20 breaths. You can initially begin with 5 to 10 breaths and gradually increase it to the former count

- Open your eyes slowly. Say that you love your baby and that you will do everything to make it happy and healthy

Caution - Do not take more than three deep breaths during your pregnancy, especially in the advanced stage.

For best results, practice this technique in the early morning, especially on your off days/ weekends! Don't forget to call the 'daddy to be' to join you while you meditate!

Is taking supplements such as Women's Health Drink (which are commercially available) good?

I would answer your question with a simple yes. However, being a holistic health practitioner I would suggest all of my clients go for natural foods and pregnancy supplements (the calcium/ iron/ DHA supplements your gynecologist prescribes).

The food and nutrition in your pregnancy very much determine your child's mental and physical health in its later years.

I would like you to consider the following in your pregnancy nutrition:

1. Take the prescribed supplements on time. And ensure your calcium and hemoglobin levels are kept normal all through the nine months

2. Drink ANTIBIOTIC FREE MILK. You can prepare dishes out of milk too.

3. Consume fresh fruits and vegetables daily

Why do periods stop during a pregnancy?

Because a woman's body needs "that blood" to sustain the life in her pregnant uterus! A female's body prepares for pregnancy every month with a layer of blood and a heap of hormones. This is similar to making a bed and other amenities for your loved ones when they arrive! When fertilization doesn't take place, the uterus cleanses itself by shedding those unwanted 'decorations'. On the other hand, if pregnancy occurs, the body builds on a lot of stuff in addition to the blood and hormones instead of menstruating!

Is it normal to have pelvic pain at 28 weeks pregnant?

Yes, it is normal. Let's see why pelvic pain is considered normal during pregnancy. But before that let me assume you are otherwise healthy and that you have no risks such as premature labor or arthritis or any other systemic or metabolic disorders.

1. The relaxing effect of hormones

As you near your term, your body prepares you for the child's birth. This is characterized by softening of your joints and ligaments! Hence you experience pain.

2. Your baby's descent

Same as the reason I have mentioned above, with the progression of your pregnancy, your baby begins to descend down into the pelvic cavity. This will create pressure in the pelvic region causing pain.

3. Incorrect posture

Incorrect posture while standing or lying down during the advanced stages of pregnancy will also put you at risk of developing pelvic pain. The reason is the altered skeletal system you have during the pregnancy.

4. Non-pregnancy causes

These include a history of the injured pelvis or existing back pain/ pelvic plain

Can pregnant women eat lalmohan/rasgulla?

Yes, they can!

But avoid the preserved ones. You might pose the risk of infection from the bottled/preserved foods.

As long as you don't suffer from Diabetes/Gestational Diabetes, you can savor the rasgullas and enjoy your good times of pregnancy! Make sure you eat sweets in moderation though!! :D You can include a lot of flavor varieties of your like during your pregnancy! Let your baby know about your pleasure when you eat those foods!

After how many days does a pregnant woman start to feel nausea?

It depends on a lot of factors, including your family history! It is usually observed from the 6th week of pregnancy. But can very well fluctuate as an early or late symptom. If vomiting or morning sickness is strong among your family members, you will have more chances of having it earlier! You are less likely to have an early morning sickness after your first pregnancy.

There are women who do not experience vomiting at all during their pregnancy. So you don't have to eagerly wait for the 'vomiting' episodes to arrive if you do not have vomiting during the pregnancy time!

What causes low appetite during early pregnancy?

Pregnancy is characterized by a lot of changes in a woman's body. She can experience low appetite due to:

1. Hormonal changes

2. Tiredness due to morning sickness

3. Difficulty adapting to the new period in her life Feeling fullness or bloating due to hormonal changes and reduced physical activity and exercise regimen (due to fear of loss of baby)

What can a low appetite cause if you overlook it?

Early pregnancy is a very crucial period as the embryo (early life form) undergoing rapid growth requires essential nutrients for the formation of its organs though in the primitive form.

Consuming food below your calorie requirement will predispose you to:

- Lethargy or tiredness to perform daily activities
- Depression and guilt due to fear of damaging the fetal life Inability to complete daily goals in household chores or office work, which again lead to the feeling of insufficiency or incomplete feeling
- Worsening of morning sickness, fainting, cramps, and other symptoms/issues that may arise during pregnancy
- Risk of developmental issues in the newborn

How dangerous are spicy cravings during pregnancy?

It is not dangerous dear Mommy! The only thing is you just have to keep moderation! Let's have a quick look at the reason why you are advised to stay away from spicy foods during pregnancy.

1. Worsens heartburn and regurgitation

During pregnancy, the muscle (sphincter) which closes your stomach relaxes. This predisposes you to heartburn and regurgitation. When you consume spicy food, imagine how you would feel if those spicy contents came up and burned your food pipe! That's painful mommy!

2. Mood changes

Consuming spicy foods can predispose you to have negative emotions such as anger, guilt, and depression. And it can affect your baby's mental coding as well as your thoughts very much affect your baby. The point is not to go overboard consuming spices during your childbearing period.

How can you cope with the craving?

The more you suppress your pregnancy craving, the more it will stress you up. Hence, rather than complete abstinence.

1. Consume spices in moderation

2. Always supplement foods such as curd, vegetable salad, and fruits every time you go for a spicy course. Ensure you drink plenty of water each day

3. Practice meditation and relaxation techniques if you feel nervous or down.

Remember, whatever you eat, eat happily!

In addition to taking prenatal vitamins, what are the best things I can do to get my body ready to conceive?

Preparing for conception is the best gift the parents can give their baby to be born!

1. Watch your weight!

Ensure both of you are in good health and stay in shape with an ideal BMI while you plan for your pregnancy. Make sure both the partners practice a daily exercise routine for at least 20 minutes.

2. Keep an eye on your habits Avoid junk foods.

Abstain from alcohol, smoking, or drugs. Stop your contraception pills at least 3 months before planning pregnancy.

3. Focus on foods you eat

Eat healthy foods rich in Zinc and Omega 3 fatty acids. Resorting to a cleaning diet or a detox diet during the planning phase of your pregnancy (within a year) could be greatly beneficial. if you feel positive, you can carry forward that healthy diet for yourself and your partner.

How soon does morning sickness start after pregnancy?

Morning sickness or nausea and vomiting during pregnancy affect over 50% of pregnancies.

What causes this sickness?

Well, the possible reasons are:

- Hormonal changes
- Neurological factors
- Psychological adjustments
- Or a combination of the above

How can you get rid of this?

Briefing some of the effective methods for tackling morning sickness

- Eating a cracker or dry biscuit with a drink before rising in the morning
- Avoidance of spicy or pungent odors and eating little and often
- Having a small number of fluids between meals to get rid of dehydration

Other conjunct therapies for Morning Sickness:

You can consider the following complementary therapies which are proven to be effective:

- Acupuncture
- Homeopathy
- Herbal remedies
- Neuro-electric stimulation

What are the risks of using x-rays during pregnancy?

The risks would be the same as that of exposing a cute flower to the burning Sun!

X-rays are notorious for changing the cell structures in a living organism. And the more delicate the cell forms are, the more risk they (the cells) possess in terms of damage!

The extent of damage can range from birth defects to fetal death depending on how powerful the exposure has been!

However, I have seen a lot of people (my co-workers) who delivered healthy babies even when they were getting exposed to radiation. They followed healthcare guidelines at our hospitals while at work and took great care of themselves during their pregnancies. Let me also tell you that the radiation they got exposed to was not that powerful.

To conclude, stay away from not only the X-rays but from direct Sun and excess hot and cold climates during pregnancy!

Is it okay to work while pregnant?

Yes, it is, provided you have not been advised strict bed rest and do not possess risk factors:

You got an added advantage when you work! Your baby too participates in your thinking process and hence you don't have to take an extra effort to help boost your baby's intelligence when it is born! But take care you give proper care in the following when you work:

- Adequate food for you and your baby (inside you)
- Proper hydration
- At least 15 minutes of physical activity (pregnancy workouts or simple walks) daily
- Manage your stress during your work

What do fetal movements feel like at 9 months pregnant?

It resembles more of a kind of newborn baby!

Yes, by the time you are 9 months pregnant, your baby would have developed almost all of its organs including lungs! if you want to know more about its capabilities, read on:

- Your baby will develop a pattern of sleep and waking It can play and move all of its body!
- Your baby now listens and recognizes its daddy's and mommy's voice.
- It can even respond to external sounds!
- You will feel the kicks are stronger by this time!

What are the stages of pregnancy?

Let's review pregnancy as 3 trimesters, each trimester comprising of 3months.

1. The first trimester

Welcome to the world of dilemmas and roller coaster rides of mood swings and nausea! Haha! I didn't really mean to scare you out. So if you're, I'm sorry! You will experience a whole lot of new sensations, mood swings, and body changes during this period. Your baby too is undergoing drastic cell division to assume an image resembling you or your partner!

2. Second trimester

You will gain weight, and your tummy will grow so as your breasts and other areas! You will be familiar with all those 'kicks' from the inside by now. In fact, by this time, you would have accepted that finally 'you are pregnant!!

3. Third trimester

You master to do all work with the full tummy just like a superwoman! A waddling gait would be common for you at this time, so you may accept and walk gracefully. You will now realize the baby now has started to respond to your as well as the daddy's voice. And as and when your due date approaches, you know all those stages have been so precious!!!

How can I treat mild cramps at 6 weeks pregnant?

Cramps can be troublesome in your pregnancy period, especially when you get in the middle of something! Give you some simple tips to alienate yourself from the 'cramp'!

1. Adequate nutrition - Ensure you take a good amount of calcium and magnesium-rich foods. I highly recommend my clients to go for foods that are culturally practiced since your elder one's times.

2. Practice exercises - Practicing leg and foot exercises several times a day will not only save you from cramps at this earlier stage but, will also enhance your lower limb (leg) circulation as and when your pregnancy advances!

3. Practice good postures - It is highly recommended that you avoid high heels and at the same time, try practicing pelvic tilts whenever you stand.

4. Stay far from the medicines - Unless and until it is prescribed by a health care practitioner, do not resort to any form of muscle relaxants/pain killers or hot massages (especially if you're on anticoagulant therapy4. Stay far from the medicines - Unless and until it is prescribed by a health care practitioner, do not resort to any form of muscle relaxants/pain killers or hot massages (especially if you're on anticoagulant therapy).

What is the maximum age to get pregnant?

The human body is just like any other living being! It undergoes natural wear and tears. When compared to a machine, the human body, as and when it gets old, loses its productivity! The best evidence is menopause, where the ovulation ceases and the woman is no longer capable of reproduction.

Hence it is wise to conceive at an age less than 35 years if you are a woman and 40 years in the case of men.

There are several reported incidences of complications and genetic disorders (especially mental retardation or

Down syndrome) in babies born to elder couples.

Again this can be a matter of debate when someone who has been into health and fitness tries for conception through a partner of excellent mental and physical health like her even at the age I have mentioned above! Moreover, with the improved living condition, both the genders bear the advantage of childbearing even at a later phase mentioned above. I have personally known and assisted couples through diet and emotional counseling during their pregnancy journey during their 40s.

Why does a woman's water break before giving birth?What is water?

The water which we refer to here is the amniotic fluid which is enclosed in a sac called an Amniotic sac. The 'water' serves as the following during pregnancy:-

- Protects the baby by acting as a shock absorber if the mommy falls or hits somewhere
- Providing optimum temperature for the baby
- The baby will also have a number of other benefits such as developing its digestive system as it goes on swallowing the fluid in addition to giving the young one a 'play ground' to flex and extend its body smoothly!

So how does it break?

it's a simple story!

As the labor progresses, the uterine muscles begin to contract to expel the baby (inside the amniotic sac filled with the 'water'). As a result, it starts to move downwards into the cervix and then the vagina. The mentioned processes build up the pressure in the sac and eventually rupture. Your Doctor can also make the water break if your labor is delayed. In that case, we call it Artificial Rupture.

What is the reason for chest pain during pregnancy?

Before answering the question, I assume you are otherwise a healthy person with no known cardiovascular disease or you're not a person with a family history of the same!

Now back to the question!

Pregnant women experience chest pain due to several changes in their bodies that they undergo during the pregnancy. Would like to throw light on two main causes:

1. Changes in the alimentary canal

During pregnancy, the sphincter (or the muscle layer) around the opening of your stomach relaxes. This makes you prone to regurgitation and heartburn. Most pregnant women report chest discomfort due to excessive gas formation too.

2. Your raising tummy

Though you will be excited to see that tummy growing up, you may or may not chest discomfort because of the reason that your enlarging uterus. It will push up the diaphragm further up resulting in a congested feeling and hence chest pain.

How do you keep a woman you love happy while she is pregnant?

When you keep your lady happy, you are designing a kid who will tend to stay happier in his/her adult life. I would like to suggest some of the tips for you:

1. Physical assurance

Your partner needs a lot of physical help from your side right from helping her in taking short walks to anything and everything you believe you could help her with! Your physical presence will secure her motherly feelings and help her stay strong during pregnancy!

2. Taking care of her food and nutrition

Pregnancy is well known for those never-ending vomiting episodes, tiredness, fainting, and the list goes on! It is very crucial that you take an active part in paying attention to what she eats! Remember, her food habits even influence your kid's later life! Moreover, she will feel blessed if she comes to know that she got someone to rely on in this 'precious time'!

3. Have fun!

Women go through a lot of emotional and physical changes during their pregnancy. This predisposes her to have stress during this time. Well, you got work here daddy, take her out to her favorite places or simply have fun with any kind of games or dance which are safe for her!

4. Say yes to sex

While most male partners feel reluctant to have sex during pregnancy for the fear of causing harm to the baby, several kinds of research show that it is absolutely safe to get intimate with your lady! (But of course, there are certain conditions such as the premature cervix, placenta previa, etc which demand abstinence from intercourse during the gestational period). Some mommies feel a higher surge of hormones during this time which makes them go wild in bed. Go with her with no worries, after all, your question is all about making her happy, isn't it! Are peanuts good for pregnant women? Absolutely good! Provided you're not allergic to it.

5. Is peanut good for women?

It is. Provided you are not allergic to it.

Peanuts are the excellent yet cheapest source of protein and folate! It helps your baby develop a good brain and ensures its proper spinal development during the initial stage of your pregnancy.

It's a good idea to have boiled or roasted peanuts as your snacks! If you eat Indian food, add them while you prepare breakfasts such as Pulav and Poha or even in your dosa batter (after grinding them). There are other delicious recipes such as peanut cutlets and vadas as well. If you wish to savor 'sweetness' instead, go grab a peanut candy!

Why do I crave soda during pregnancy?

Not only Soda, but I bet there are a whole lot of funny likes you might develop when you're expecting. This can be due to the psychological or hormonal changes in your body.

Giving some of the facts to consider while you crave soda:

1. The carbonated water will enlarge your stomach. During pregnancy, the tight muscle closing your stomach (cardiac sphincter) loosens up causing heartburn and regurgitation. Drinking carbonated water can worsen the situation as your pregnancy progresses
2. The carbonated sugary drink contains a lot of sugar in it! It will not only burden your body to sweep away the excess sugar but can prove detrimental to your young one too.
3. If you have Gestational Diabetes, stay way clear of this dangerous drink!
4. Drinking soda will never satiate your thirst resulting in you gulping down a lot more fluid than the required amount. This can disturb your sleep as you might feel an urgency to urinate.

How can you cope?

- Well, you can try a plain soda rather than a sweetened version initially. Gradually bring it down.

- Practice meditation and interesting workouts will help deviate your mind to some extent.
- The healthy alternatives are fruit juice or smoothies

Can I get pregnant on 21 days of my period? Where do I have a cycle of 28 days?

Here's a simple calendar with which you can plan your pregnancy.

Simultaneously you can rely on the mucus secretion you are more likely to have when you ovulate. This period would also be a 'fertile period' for you.

Make sure that both of you (you and your partner) are in good health (both mentally and physically) when you plan for your pregnancy!

Is it more dangerous to be pregnant if you are overweight?

If you're overweight, your chances of conception are less when compared to a woman with ideal body weight. The same goes for men as well. Men's BMI also determines their chances of getting pregnant.

Being overweight during pregnancy predisposes you to a number of conditions starting from developing gestational diabetes to a number of other illnesses which I wouldn't tell you because I don't intend to scare you out!

You will gain an extra 12 to 13 Kilogram body weight during your pregnancy. You might feel you are thus feeling 'heavy'.

Having put on body weight, it is difficult to take breaths when you walk for a while. As the pregnancy progresses, your growing uterus will raise your diaphragm further up, which will congest your lungs making your pregnancy period an unpleasant one (in cases where you feel breathless. There are women who undergo pregnancy with ease, so do not panic!)

Exercises are very important during your pregnancy as it helps strengthen your pelvic muscle for your labor. If you are obese, you will have problems performing the 'push' for your baby to come out.

To conclude, the 'overweight phenomenon is common during pregnancy. It is important to have a healthy diet and a healthy mind during this time. Working out will help you stay safer during and after your pregnancy. If you observe drastic weight gain, consult your Physician and get the advice for its management.

References

1. National Library of Medicine: https://www.ncbi.nlm.nih.gov/books/NBK560395/
2. Mayo Clinic: https://www.mayoclinic.org/
3. World Health Organization: https://www.who.int/
4. Hiralal Konar, DC Dutta's textbook of Obstetrics, 8th Edition, Jaypee Publication
5. Diane M Fraser, Margaret A Cooper, Myles' Textbook for Midwives, 14th Edition, Elsevier Publication
6. Pictures and Photos: Google and Unsplash